The Soul of Wellness

The Soul of Wellness

*12 Holistic Principles for
Achieving a Healthy Body,
Mind, Heart, and Spirit*

Rajiv Parti, M.D.

SelectBooks, Inc.
New York

This book is meant as a source of information only. The information should by no means replace the advice of your personal medical professional who should always be consulted when beginning any new regimen of diet or exercise or entering a program for treatment of physical pain, or treatment for conditions of addictions, treatment for depression or other psychological distress, or for treatment of any other medical condition. Your personal medical professional should always be consulted before pursuing any alternative medicine health treatment program or any alternative medicines recommended for general physical or mental health or the treatment of any specific health conditions or illness. The author and publisher expressly disclaim responsibility for any adverse effects resulting from following the use or application of information contained herein.

This edition published by SelectBooks, Inc.
For information address SelectBooks, Inc., New York, New York.

First Edition

ISBN 978-1-59079-955-0

Cataloging-in-Publication Data

Parti, Rajiv.
  The soul of wellness : 12 holistic principles for achieving a healthy
body, mind, heart, and spirit / Rajiv Parti. -- 1st ed.
    p. cm.
  Summary: "Former Chief of Anesthesiology at Bakersfield Heart Hospital and founder of the Pain Management Institute of California emerges from healing his own chronic pain and severe depression following a personal health crisis to advocate 12 holistic principles of wellness based on Eastern spiritual practices"-- Provided by publisher.
  ISBN 978-1-59079-955-0 (pbk. : alk. paper)
  1. Holistic medicine--Popular works. 2. Mind and body therapies--Popular works. 3. Self-care, Health--Popular works. I. Title.
  R733.R34 2012
  613--dc23
                      2012020158

Manufactured in the United States of America

10 9 8 7 6 5 4 3 2 1

CONTENTS

PREFACE

CS

An Adventure into Wellness

To seek out and discover the fundamental principles of wellness can be an exciting adventure, one that affects all aspects of our lives. It is an adventure that includes coming to understand the power of Spirit to help us achieve maximum wellness in all dimensions. That is what this book is about—how Spirit can become a profound source of healing, harmony, and happiness for each of us. Before we begin this adventure, it may help you to better understand the roots of this book if I tell you a few things about myself and my own journey into wellness.

I always wanted to be a healer. But as a boy, I was unsure of what kind. Sometimes I leaned toward medicine, having a close relative who was a physician. At other times, I thought spirituality was my calling. I pondered deep questions: Why are we here? What is the purpose of life? I even seriously considered becoming a monk.

In time, though, I decided my calling was medicine. I earned my M.D. degree from Delhi University and in 1982 emigrated to the United States, where I took advanced training in anesthesiology. I became a successful practicing anesthesiologist and specialist in pain management. In 1987 I married my beautiful wife and best friend, and we had three wonderful children.

I eventually became Chief of Anesthesiology at a large community hospital. Life was good. I was fulfilling the American dream materialistically, with a large house and expensive cars. Then two crucial factors entered my life.

The first was growing dissatisfaction as I realized that making money was not the key to my happiness. I began to again ask those questions from childhood: What gives life its greatest meaning? What is the source of happiness? The second factor was a serious wrist injury that threatened my work. Several surgeries failed to solve the problem, and I developed reflex sympathetic dystrophy. This resulted in chronic pain in my wrist, arm, and shoulder. I was taking pain medications but not getting better. I decided to try alternative pain management therapies and began a program of regular meditation and visualization. The results were very positive. I was able to continue doing the work I loved. These two factors wakened in me a great interest in mind-body medicine and the science of happiness and fulfillment. I began studying scientific research in the field and spoke to key people such as Deepak Chopra, M.D., Dr. David Frawley, and Robin Sharma. I attended a mind-body course at Harvard Medical School. I began understanding that wellness is multi-dimensional, encompassing physical, psychological, social, and spiritual well-being, and that the science of wellness should include both scientific research and ancient wisdom. The word "healer" took on a new meaning for me. I realized that I want to be a healer not only of the body, but of the mind and spirit.

I had just started writing about and speaking on total wellness when I discovered I had prostate cancer, and my Dark Night of the Soul began. I underwent surgery for the cancer, but there were complications. Then there were further surgeries and more complications. On Christmas Eve, 2010, I developed a severe post-surgery infection. Shivering like a leaf, with a 105-degree temperature, I was rushed to the hospital thinking I would die. The infection was drained and finally defeated, but I was left with raw, open surgical wounds for weeks after. All of these complications left me physically, psychologically, socially, and spiritually drained.

But my Dark Night continued. I developed chronic pelvic pain from the half dozen urological surgeries I had undergone, as well as severe depression. I was on a combination of anti-depressants and pain meds. Because I was technically physically well with medication, I was deemed well enough to go back to work as an anesthesiologist. But I knew it was not the right thing to do because even a slight error in my judgment could kill somebody, and given all the medications I was on, that slight error seemed possible. I wouldn't do it. I therefore found myself unable to work and having to go on medical disability. My income dropped precipitously and I had to sell my house at a substantial loss and move to one a quarter the price of my previous house. I had lost my job, my income, my house, all that was—at least superficially—dear to me. It was as if one-by-one the lights were switching off.

But the dearest thing of all I did not lose—my family. My wife's true, unconditional love was my anchor during this emotional tsunami. Due to her love and support and that of the rest of my family, as well as the harmonious balancing effects of Ayurveda and my focusing more and more on spiritual principles, my Dark Night finally passed.

Today, I am well again in all dimensions. But I had to face that long trial to reconfirm and solidify my true purpose. Though I could now return to being an anesthesiologist, it is time for me to go much further. I now aspire to be a healer of all dimensions, while emphasizing the power of Spirit and the underlying spirituality that connects us all. I speak now as a medical doctor who also personally understands the trials of a patient. As a physician, I want to dwell in the Science of Happiness and the medical benefits of ancient traditions like meditation, yoga, and Ayurveda.

You are holding in your hands some of the fruits of my latest efforts to understand and transmit the principles of wellness. *The Soul of Wellness* is about the very essence of well-being—Spirit. It explains some of the many ways Spirit can enter into our lives, empowering us and creating greater wellness in all dimensions of our existence.

Let us begin our adventure into wellness as we explore together its deepest principles.

ACKNOWLEDGMENTS

I want to express my sincere appreciation to some very important people in my life and to some special people who provided crucial input as *The Soul of Wellness* was being completed. First of all, I want to thank my mother Swaran Parti, and my father J.C. Parti, for their indelible love and unwavering support throughout my life. You raised me as all parents should raise their children—to believe I was capable of doing anything I set my mind and hard work to. Thank you from the bottom of my heart, Mom and Dad.

To my beautiful and inspiring wife, Arpana, and my three wonderful children; thank you so much for standing strong and close with me these many years. Thank you most of all just for being who you are and for bringing your precious and always wondrous reality into my life. I love you all more than I can say.

To write and publish a book such as *The Soul of Wellness* requires the diligent work of a number of people. I am grateful to the staff at Select-Books for their dedication to bringing this book to fruition, and am especially appreciative of my publisher Kenzi Sugihara for his professionalism and for smoothing out the entire process. To my personal assistant Rakhi Kumar, I want to thank you again and again for your astute and ever-perceptive support as the publication process progressed, as well as both before and after. And finally, I want to offer a very special thank-you to my friend and editor, Harvey McCloud, Ph.D., for helping me find the words to best express my ideas about spirituality and wellness, as well as for offering his own substantial knowledge and insights to *The Soul of Wellness* as it was being completed. His efforts have been pivotal every step of the way.

ය

Defining the Soul of Wellness

W*ellness* is something we hear a lot about these days. We all know the term denotes something very desirable, something we should be seeking. But what, actually, is wellness?

Some might say that wellness refers to physical health and leave it at that. But how about people who are mostly physically healthy, but also very stressed out, lonely, fearful, or unhappy? Do these people have wellness? Not totally. They may have a degree of physical well-being, but not complete wellness. That's because wellness includes much more than physiological health. In fact, wellness has four dimensions, each one essential to your overall well-being and satisfaction with life.

Three Dimensions of Wellness: Body, Mind, and Heart

Three of the four dimensions of wellness are widely accepted today. The first dimension is *Body*. This includes all aspects of your physical health—your cardiovascular system, immune system, and all the rest. To have *Wellness of Body,* all of these systems must be working together in an efficient, natural way.

Physical wellness is crucial because your body is one of your two fundamental instruments for living. It is through your body that you are able to see and smell the beauty of a rose and hear the lilting call of a bird. It is by means of your body that you can stroll through a park, refinish a bookcase, and change a diaper to insure the cleanliness of your baby.

The healthier your body, the better you are able to perceive the world around you and perform a thousand important functions each day.

The second dimension of wellness is *Mind,* your other fundamental instrument for living. Your mind consists of a cognitive (thinking) part and an affective (feeling) part. The cognitive part includes your beliefs, thoughts, and imaginings. Through this aspect of your mind, when it is whole and functioning well, you are able to make sense of your experiences, communicate with others, and plan for your future. The affective part includes your emotions, motivations, and attitudes toward life. This aspect of your mind, when it is healthy, enables you to enjoy a beautiful sunset, feel empathy for a friend, and get excited about a new project. *Wellness of Mind* encompasses both parts of your mind. It includes thinking clearly, taking a positive approach to the world, and finding interest and joy in the world around you. Wellness of Mind is essential for living a happy life steeped in rich, rewarding experiences.

The third dimension of wellness is *Heart.* This dimension consists of your capacity to have good relationships with other people and to do so with generosity and understanding. I use the word "Heart" because traditionally, we think of the heart as the source of our caring for others. It is Heart that takes you out to lunch with a friend, cares for a child who is ill, and enjoys a barbecue with your neighbors. *Wellness of Heart* includes spending quality time with family and friends. It also means showing kindness to others and concern for those less fortunate than you. There is ample reason to believe that happiness and overall well-being depend on living a life with Heart as much as they do on physical and mental health.

These three dimensions of wellness—Body, Mind, and Heart—are three pillars upon which we build our lives. But unlike most pillars, they do not stand totally separate from each other. In fact, they are very much interrelated.

Take the relationship of Body to Mind. We all know that having a bad cold can slow our thinking processes and create emotional boredom. And we know that a good cardiovascular workout can make us mentally sharper and give us an emotional boost. These are just two examples of the countless ways Wellness of Body can affect Wellness of Mind. Similarly, Mind affects Body; Heart affects Mind, and so on through all the combinations. When we create wellness in any of these three dimensions, we promote wellness in the others. The relationship isn't perfect, of course.

We can be rich in Mind and relatively poor in Body, or rich in Body and poor in the relationships that constitute Heart. But in general, an increase in wellness in any dimension helps increase wellness in the others.

This interrelatedness of Body, Mind, and Heart makes it even clearer that to enjoy a rich and satisfying sojourn on Earth—a life full of meaningful relationships, activities, and pleasures—we need maximum wellness in all three dimensions.

Spirit as the Fourth Dimension of Wellness

Most people today recognize the importance of these first three dimensions of wellness. But there is one more dimension that many people barely recognize. Yet this fourth dimension of wellness is as important as the other three for living a happy and fulfilling life. In fact, it is so fundamental that it forms the core, the essence, the very *Soul* of Wellness.

The fourth dimension of wellness I am talking about is *Spirit.*

Spirit is about feeling connected to something much larger than ourselves, something precious, enduring, and of infinite value. For some, the spiritual connection consists of a felt relationship to a Creator or a Higher Reality. Others feel a sacred connection to the natural world or to humanity. For still others, dedication to perennial values such as truth and compassion guide their lives. Embracing our spiritual dimension in any of these ways creates meaning and promotes *Wellness of Spirit.* This spiritual wellness:

- Helps us make sense of our lives

- Opens us to the goodness and beauty surrounding us

- Gives us a deep appreciation for the world, other people, and ourselves

- Releases the Divinity that resides within us.

Despite its importance, many in today's society have lost sight of this fourth dimension of wellness. Even if they attend religious services or occasionally contemplate the wonder and mystery of existence, these experiences play little part in their daily activities. As a result, they lack the powerful sense of meaning and depth that comes from fully engaging their spiritual dimension. They also miss out on the synergistic power of Spirit to infuse and promote wellness in the other three dimensions of their lives.

Part of the problem may be that people don't understand how Spirit can help create overall well-being. It is easy to comprehend how wellness in Body promotes wellness in Mind and how good relationships (Heart) make us feel better physically and mentally. But it may not be clear how wellness of Spirit can promote our well-being in the other dimensions. Yet spiritual wellness can profoundly affect Body, Mind, and Heart. One way it does this is by clarifying what is truly important to us.

Emily's Journey to a More Spiritual Understanding through Yoga and Meditation

As an example, consider Emily, a successful businesswoman with a husband and two school-aged girls.

Physically, Emily seemed to have plenty of energy and appeared to be healthy. Mentally, her challenging work kept her sharp. And socially, she was active outside the home, while she also tried to provide quality time to her husband and daughters.

A casual observer might have concluded that Emily was on top of things in regard to Body, Mind, and Heart. But actually, she was less well in those dimensions than she appeared. A main reason was her recent promotion to a more responsible position, which had resulted in a lot of job-related stress. This had led to a rise in her blood pressure and a peptic ulcer. The pressure was also taking a mental toll. She was enjoying her work much less than before, and stress headaches often made it difficult for her to think clearly. Socially, too, things were not as satisfactory as they seemed. Though Emily had many acquaintances, she had no close friends. And most of the events she attended were job-related and gave her little joy. At home, she tried hard to give time to her husband and girls, but worrying about problems at work often made her irritable and distant.

In the face of these issues, Emily had begun questioning her life. She would lie awake at night wondering: Why don't I enjoy things more? Why am I working so hard? What's the purpose of my life, anyway, just to keep making money until I die?

In the midst of this increasingly disturbing and chaotic situation, Emily's aerobics instructor invited her to attend a yoga class. Yoga? Emily thought. Isn't that something only people who are interested in Eastern religions do? But when the instructor mentioned that yoga was a good stress reliever, she decided to give it a try.

The yoga teacher, a mature woman, was very competent. As she led the classes, she exuded calmness and wisdom. Emily quickly found that yoga did in fact relax her physically and mentally. Soon, she began staying after class to talk with the teacher about the history and philosophy of yoga. She starting feeling that an entire world of Spirit was opening up to her. When she discovered that the instructor also taught a class in meditation, she immediately joined. As she learned the ancient art of meditation, she was amazed at how it alleviated her stressful feelings and opened her mind.

When she meditated, she became acutely aware of herself and her surroundings. She would feel herself at the center of a sometimes challenging, but ultimately loving universe that included her husband, children, co-workers, and clients. At home, she started reading the Bible, a book she had not opened since she was a child. There she found many passages that made beautiful sense to her. Her questions about life began resolving themselves. Gradually, she came to see the meaning of her life as centered on simply loving and helping to provide for her family, striving to be a sharp but compassionate businessperson, and enjoying being alive each moment of the day.

In short, Emily began acquiring Wellness of Spirit. As a result, she found her wellness improving in the other three dimensions. At work, problems stopped aggravating and worrying her so much. She could sometimes even laugh at a problematic situation as she set about tackling it. At home she was more engaged with her kids and husband and was no longer short with them. And two months after she started the meditation class, she found that her blood pressure had dropped back to normal and her ulcer was virtually gone.

Emily's story is not unusual. Again and again I have seen individuals whose wellness was being compromised in Body, Mind, and Heart because they paid little attention to the dimension of Spirit. In some cases, the person eventually went into a tailspin that led to addictive behaviors, depression, financial ruin, divorce, or even suicide. In other, happier cases, the individual managed to pull out of their descent before it was too late. For most if not all of the second group, the pull-out came when they opened up their spiritual dimension.

How do I know this? Because I have been there. Years ago, I found myself in a terrible tailspin at a time when my spiritual wellness was very low. What brought me out of the turmoil was Spirit working through the love of my family. Later, as I learned more about the fundamental principles of spiritual wellness, I began to soar to new heights of well-being in all dimensions of my life. And that's why I am writing this book—to help others soar.

Throughout humankind's existence, Spirit has been greatly needed, and our time is no exception. Today we face a powerful challenge to our spiritual dimension—unbridled egoism and runaway materialism. As technology brings material comforts and affluence to millions of people, the desire to gain more and more possessions has become ascendant in many societies.

It is not that money and ownership are bad. On the contrary, money can purchase many fine things—a comfortable home, educational opportunities, travel, freedom from drudgery, and much more. In fact, if used wisely, money can help foster Spirit in the world. The problem is the idea that making as much money as possible is the most worthwhile goal in life. When this idea becomes dominant in a person's mind, it often quickly breeds another idea—the belief that it is all right to make money in any way available. And it is these two ideas—that nothing has more value than money and that it is acceptable to make money *at all other costs*—that make up the unhealthy core of runaway materialism.

This extreme materialism has a stranglehold on countless people in our society. For some, it seems to be a death grip. People who already have many things are unhappy because they want more—getting more is the only thing that ever truly motivates them. People who don't have as much are unhappy because others have more. And they remain dissatisfied as long as affluence eludes them.

This constant focus on making money and acquiring possessions amounts to a rejection of Spirit. This is a tragedy on many levels. Spirit is so vast, so deep and important, that it should infuse our lives on a daily basis. It is through Spirit that we perceive the majesty of a mountain, the blessedness in a child's laughter, and the magic in a firefly's tiny light. It is through Spirit that we come to understand that we are unique and have a holy purpose in life. It is through Spirit that we find meaning in our day-to-day work, our relationships with others, and our perceptions of the world.

Some may think that to embrace Spirit in their lives it is enough to spend an hour a week in a church, temple, or mosque, or a few minutes contemplating nature or the stars. But if they ignore their spiritual dimension for the rest of the week, they are effectively disavowing Spirit.

Those who turn their backs on Spirit fail to recognize it as a critically important dimension of their lives. The idea of spiritual wellness never occurs to them. They also fail to recognize that by ignoring wellness in Spirit, they are sabotaging their wellness in Body, Mind, and Heart. Like Emily, it is essential for each of us to understand who we are within a larger context. The questions that Emily found herself facing are questions we all can ask. Who am I in relation to my family and friends, humanity, and nature? What purpose should I seek in life? How should I approach each day? What should I strive to leave behind when I die? These are questions of Spirit. And the answers we find to those questions will have an immense bearing on our wellness in all dimensions of our being.

In fact, without Spirit, total wellness in any dimension is impossible to achieve. This is most obvious for Heart. Without Spirit, Heart degenerates into cold, uncaring relationships lacking in kindness and respect. For millions of people, such relationships are the norm. Without Spirit, the dimension of Heart has no heart.

This is because Spirit is the wellspring of love. Consider a mother cradling her baby in her arms, cherishing and protecting the little child. There is nothing more full of Spirit than the mother's actions at that moment. And there is nothing more full of Heart. The two go hand in hand. Spirit infuses the Heart with love, and we carry that love to our relationships with others. Without Spirit, there is no true Heart and no wellness of Heart.

Without Spirit, total wellness also eludes Mind. If we ignore Spirit and get caught in the grip of unrestrained ego-gratification, our thoughts and imaginings revolve around what we can get for ourselves and how to get it. Our emotions are dominated by selfishness and greed. Our motivations are totally self-serving as we consider other people to be mere tools for our use. We are willing to twist the truth like a pretzel to serve our own interests. Those who allow themselves to be dominated by a grasping ego usually believe that their ideas and behavior are in their best interest. But they could not be more wrong. Behavior dominated by such drives does not bring happiness. Instead, it promotes a shallow, self-serving life without depth, without caring relationships, without honor. It eventually fosters anxiety, alienation, loneliness, and depression—the opposite of emotional wellness.

But if we embrace Spirit, nourishing beliefs take root and then blossom in our minds. We come to understand the holiness of the world and every person in it. We begin thinking deeply about the purpose of our lives and what undertakings have greatest value for us. We develop beliefs about the importance of living in the truth and about being open to the goodness of the world. Such beliefs are the epitome of wellness in the thinking part of Mind. As for the feeling part, Spirit infuses us with positive emotions, attitudes, and motivations that reveal life to us as it truly is and can be. We begin feeling the world as an infinite garden of delight, beauty, and possibility.

Even in the case of Body, total wellness is impossible without Spirit. Emily is a good example of this. The positive values and meanings brought by Spirit help to defuse the anxieties created by modern life. They heal the physiological ravages of stress. A strong spiritual outlook strengthens the immune system and fosters resilience. Spirit also teaches us that Body is holy. This is a powerful motivator for taking care of ourselves physically. If we allow it to do so, Spirit can permeate Body as completely as it does Heart and Mind.

From all of this, it is very clear that Spirit is not something that exists in some metaphysical space totally separate from us. It can infuse our lives deeply right here, right now, if we allow it to do so. It has a profound practical relationship to our well-being in all of our dimensions.

Spirit, simply put, is the *Soul of Wellness*. That is the deep truth that informs this book. In the coming pages you will learn principles and practices of Spirit that can foster wellness in each dimension of your being. Overall, you will learn from this book how to welcome Spirit into your life so that it flows clearly and deeply throughout your Body, Mind, and Heart.

Each of the following chapters focuses on some key principle that teaches us how Spirit can infuse our lives with greater meaning, direction, and wellness. From the Ayurvedic emphasis on balancing inner nature with outer nature, to the Virtues of Heart and the Blessings of Gratitude, to explaining how Spirit creates a home in each of us, these principles are designed to leap off the page, reverberate within you, and create a space where wellness can prosper. Along the way, you will learn the stories of others who have found the joyous touch of Spirit empowering their lives. At the end of the discussion of each principle you will find two exercises to provide you with an opportunity to delve deeper into the insights or to put them into practice. Think of the exercises as a kind of workbook that accompanies the lessons found in *The Soul of Wellness*.

What I most want you to take from this book is Hope, Healing, and Harmony.

Hope is your belief that you can fulfill your dreams. We all hope for a physically healthy life of accomplishment, rich experience, love, and beauty. But sometimes we may find ourselves in difficult situations when our hopes wane. At such points, renewing our Spirit can make a tremendous difference in our lives, rejuvenating hope, promoting wellness in all four dimensions, and empowering us to move into the future.

Healing is a quality that pertains to all four of our dimensions. To achieve total wellness, we must seek healing in every aspect of our being. This book focuses on the intimate relationship of our spiritual dimension to Heart, Mind, and Body. Because of this relationship, spiritual principles and practices are able to foster healing and total wellness in all four dimensions.

Finally, these pages are about increasing **Harmony** in your life. Body, Mind, Heart, and Spirit are four aspects of a single infinitely valuable being—you. When you attend to the Soul of Wellness, which is Spirit, you promote balance and harmony in all four of your dimensions. The result is a beautiful music with deep overtones that echo and reverberate throughout your life. That music is the harmony of wellness.

cs

Ayurveda

Balance Inner Nature with Outer Nature

"He who knows others is learned;
he who knows himself is wise."

Lao-Tzu
from *Tao Te Ching*

Our human bodies are exquisitely complex and functional. Consider the rapid, delicate adjustments of our eyes while reading a book or of our fingers while tying a ribbon; these and a million other physical actions are far more wondrous than the most up-to-date inventions of technology. Our bodies are also immeasurably more important than any technological gadget. A new camera or printer can be a fine tool, but it is through our physical presence that we live our lives. And if the camera or printer goes wrong, we can purchase a new one. But there are no stores that sell new bodies.

Despite this, countless people provide only lackadaisical care for this most precious instrument. Such neglect is made all too easy by the many temptations we encounter these days. The two cornerstones of healthy living, diet and exercise, face countless enticements that are contrary to the bodies that have evolved for us humans. Physiologically, we are not meant to eat supersized portions of high-calorie meals, or to sit motionless night after night in front of a television or computer. By giving into such temptations, we overwork our bodies in some ways; for example, by forcing it to digest and assimilate large amounts of fat. In other ways we underwork them by not getting enough cardiovascular or strength exercise. The result is a body out of balance.

This is why it is crucial that we understand what I call "the wisdom of healthy living." This wisdom is about how to keep our bodily systems in balance. Fortunately, information about how to maintain health is increasingly available from books, the Internet, and other sources. However, most of this information consists only of physiological strategies. It takes little account of the connections among Body, Mind, Heart, and Spirit. But the wisdom of healthy living must pay attention to these other three dimensions of our lives. In a word, it must be *holistic*. In this chapter, I will explain the basic principles of an ancient and revered health and wellness system that takes such a holistic view. It began thousands of years ago in the Far East and continues as the primary wellness resource in present-day India with its one billion people. This wellness system is called *Ayurveda*, a name combining two Sanskrit words—*ayu*, meaning life, and *veda*, meaning knowledge. Thus, the term Ayurveda means, literally, the very thing we have been talking about—the wisdom or knowledge of healthy living. I especially want to explain how the spiritual basis of this ancient wellness system can empower us to live in balance with the natural world. So, after providing a few details about Ayurveda, I will focus on the principles and practices of its spiritual foundations.

The Philosophy of Ayurveda

Ayurveda grew out of a philosophy about human nature. This philosophy holds that we are integral parts of a universe that is not only physical, but also permeated by Mind and Spirit. Because we reflect the universe in our essential nature, we too are composed of Body, Mind, and Spirit. This picture is similar to the four-dimensional view I explained in the introduction. We need only add that we are also social creatures, so Heart is yet another aspect of our being, one that is very human.

Based on this philosophy, Ayurveda began over 5,000 years ago and was passed down by word of mouth for hundreds of years. Eventually, the philosophy and the principles of Ayurveda were set down in four famous texts called the Vedas. Written about 3,500 years ago, the Rig Veda is the oldest religious text aside from certain funeral texts of the ancient Egyptians.

In its wisdom of healthy living, Ayurveda holds that at birth, we are animated by prana, a life force that exists throughout the universe. We are also infused with five basic principles that govern the universe: air, space, fire, water, and earth. These principles are inside of us in the form of various qualities that we all exhibit. For example, air and space are represented in our bodies and minds by the qualities of lightness and spaciousness. Likewise, fire is represented by the heat within our living body, water by the moisture in our body, and earth by our flesh and bones. These qualities can be combined to form three bio-energetic forces, or patterns of energy, that govern our physical constitution. The three *doshas* are:

Vata — air and space

Pitta — fire and water

Kapha — water and earth

According to Ayurveda, each dosha affects our body, mind, and spirit. In the body, the energy of Vata governs our bodily movement, perception, circulation, and respiration; the energy of Pitta governs metabolism, including digestion and absorption; and the energy of Kapha governs growth and lubrication, including bodily tissues such as muscle and fat. In the mind, Vata relates to the movement from thought to thought, Pitta helps us assimilate our thoughts to gain understanding, and Kapha enhances memory and empathy. In our spiritual aspect, Vata is manifested as the life force, Pitta determines how brilliant the life force is, and Kapha governs our ability to protect our life force, and thus our life, in the face of threats and adversity.

On the Ayurvedic view, each person is born with a unique combination of the three doshas. This combination makes up the individual's specific constitution, including his or her body type (you will learn more about this in the first exercise at the end of the chapter). Some people are primarily Vata types with fewer qualities of Pitta and Kapha. Others are mostly Pitta or Kapha. Some have two primary doshas, and a few have all three in roughly equal measure. We enter the world with each of our three doshas in perfect equilibrium. But over time, stressful impacts from outside as well as unwise personal decisions may throw our constitution out of balance, making us vulnerable to disease.

The Ayurvedic physician's purpose is first to understand the patient's unique constitution of doshas. The practitioner then determines a precise regimen of diet, sleep, and other activities that will match the patient's constitution and help maintain or restore the correct balance of the doshas. The physician understands how external forces such as herbs and massage, as well as internal forces such as meditation, can help reinstate an equilibrium that has been lost. Since mental and spiritual well-being play such an important part in health and wellness, the Ayurvedic practitioner also learns strategies

The Ayurvedic Approach to Addiction Recovery

For Ayurveda, recovery from addiction to alcohol, cigarettes, or drugs begins with the addicted person being willing to be treated. From there, it proceeds to understanding the reasons for the addiction and then undertaking several important lifestyle changes. These include an herbal-based detoxification process, practicing meditation and yoga, and going on a nutritious vegetarian diet.

Herbal therapy begins with hot herbal teas and herbal spices in food. These are intended to soothe and balance the battered digestive system. Therapy continues with an herbal detoxification process to purify the body. The original Ayurvedic cleansing process consisted of five therapies to root out deeply embedded stress and toxins and to help balance the doshas. Today, many practitioners reduce this to three therapies: Nasya (nasal cleaning), Basti (enemas), and Virechana (purgation). Ayurveda offers herbs such as Brahmi (*Bacopa monnieri*), Guduchi (*Tinospora cordifolia*), Yashtimadhu (*Glycyrrhiza glabra*), and Shankhpushpi (*Convolvulus pluricaulis*) to restore memory and cognitive function that may have been impaired by the addiction.

A strict vegetarian diet is imposed on the addicted person. This consists of cooked whole grains, fresh vegetables, and fruits. Such food is highly nutritious and contains all the required vitamins and minerals. The diet should also include ghee (clarified butter), which acts as a lubricant and strengthens the immune system.

for evaluating psychological wellness and for helping patients enhance their spiritual well-being. Overall, the goal of Ayurvedic therapies is to help people realize optimum wellness in all aspects of their existence.

While Ayurveda's sister science, Yoga, is widely practiced today in the West, Ayurveda itself is less well known. But this is changing. There is a growing appreciation for the centuries of knowledge represented by Ayurveda, and an increasing number of Westerners are learning about it as a complementary and alternative medical (CAM) system. Respected medical centers in the United States have begun embracing various aspects of Ayurveda, along with other CAM therapies. The efficacy of Ayurveda is still being evaluated in the West; however, there is growing evidence that it can be effective for many patients, especially those facing chronic illnesses such as arthritis.

Several principles of Ayurveda help explain its increasing acceptance in the West. One of these is its emphasis not on just curing disease, but on preventing it. While the Western medical model focuses on treating illness, Ayurveda gives equal importance to prevention. A second reason for the growing acceptance of Ayurveda is its holistic nature. Thousands of years ago, Ayurvedic physicians understood something that is only starting to be understood in the West—that mental, physical, and spiritual health are intertwined. This means that understanding mental and spiritual deficiencies and restoring proper balance in these areas is as important as treating physical imbalances.

A third reason Ayurveda is taking root in the West is its emphasis on the individual person. Patients of Western medicine often feel that their unique characteristics are overlooked by health practitioners. But Ayurveda insists that each of us has a unique physical and mental constitution and that a physician must understand this constitution in order to provide effective treatment. As a result, the physician is very focused on the individual. A fourth aspect of Ayurveda that many in the West find attractive is its emphasis on self-understanding and on taking personal responsibility for one's own health and wellness.

The Soul of Wellness in Ayurveda

Apart from its details, Ayurveda presents a profound spiritual vision of wellness. For Ayurveda, the idea of an isolated human being unconnected to anything else is a fiction. Each of us is intimately related to a world with countless beneficial aspects, from the sun that warms us, to the nourishing vegetables and herbs that we eat, to the bacteria that line our gastrointestinal tract and aid in digestion. But the world also includes dangers—hurricanes, poisonous mushrooms, life-threatening viruses, and many more. The wisdom of healthy living requires us to develop strategies for coexisting in harmony with this double-edged universe. We must understand how outer nature affects our inner nature. For example, which foods energize our bodies and which ones clog our arteries? Which herbs and spices sharpen our minds, and which ones dull our senses? Based on this understanding, we must balance inner nature with outer nature.

Over thousands of years Ayurveda and other nature-focused wellness systems developed much wisdom about living in harmony with nature. This was helped by the fact that communities remained small, with most people employed in jobs that involved close contact with nature. But today the percentage of people who live and work in natural settings has greatly decreased, while jobs in artificial environments have burgeoned. As a result, knowledge about how to live in harmony with nature has been forgotten by many. In this country millions of people drive each morning on clogged freeways to jobs where the natural world is represented by a potted plant or two and a few windows looking out on a smoggy sky. They then return on the same busy freeway to lodgings with very little or no green space. For these millions, nature can seem far away, as if it is in another world.

But despite appearances, even those among us who are surrounded by pavement and concrete are as fully a part of nature as people who lived a hundred or a thousand years ago. Every breath we inhale is of air that has circumvented the globe. The energy in every bite of food we ingest can ultimately be traced to some plant warmed by the sun. And though an office may be graced by only a single fern, countless other unseen denizens of the natural world are close at hand, including bacteria and viruses that can set us low.

Ayurveda's greatest gift is that it brings us back to the natural universe that we are part of. It insists that nature must be respected and embraced because it is the home into which we are born and where we *must* live. For Ayurveda, it is hopeless to seek wellness without learning how to balance our inner nature with outer nature. To try to create physical, mental, and social health without working in harmony with the world around us is like trying to breathe without air.

Mark's Change to a More Spiritual Life in Balance with Nature

This outlook is deeply spiritual in two ways. First, it puts wellness into a broad context, which is one hallmark of spirituality. Second, it holds that the universe to which we are intimately related is spiritual to its core—and therefore, so are we. One way to illustrate the double spirituality that informs Ayurveda is to tell you about a man I will call Mark.

Mark is a very modern man. He works downtown in a concrete jungle and lives in a high-rise building at the edge of the city. Several years back, unhappy with life, Mark became addicted to some of society's worst blandishments. Forty pounds overweight, he spent his evenings watching television, got little exercise, smoked a pack of cigarettes a day, and on many nights drank himself to sleep. His physician warned him that his bodily systems were gradually going haywire and that he needed to go on a diet, join a gym, and give up smoking and drinking to restore his body's natural balance. But Mark considered his addictions to be necessary evils to make his days livable. He convinced himself that as long as he kept taking his cholesterol and high blood pressure medications, everything would work out fine in the end. In reality, he was on the road to disaster.

One day, a business trip took Mark to a city close to the childhood home he had not seen in almost three decades. After his morning meeting, he was free the rest of the day, so he decided to take the hour drive to the small community where he grew up. The town, he learned on arrival, had changed little. On its outskirts, he found the house where he had been raised. It was empty and up for sale. Mark walked around to the big back yard and discovered that the area where he had grown vegetables as a child was still there. He wandered down to the stream edging the property and sat there on a big rock warmed by the spring sun.

As he listened to the murmur of the water, he thought about the many days he had enjoyed playing by the stream. Back then, it had seemed he was always outside, loving the sun, the rain and snow, and the stars at night. In his little garden he had grown tomatoes, lettuce, and watermelons. How sweet it had been to come out on a hot August day, pick a ripe tomato off the vine, and eat it right there, its juice streaming down his chin. He thought about how things had changed so radically for him since then.

As he sat brooding, he noticed a spider's web in a clump of grass near the rock. He was struck by how perfectly symmetrical it seemed. While he regarded the web, a dragonfly buzzed over his head, then back again as if to show off its iridescent pink and green wings. Then a golden butterfly passed across his line of sight. It hung in the air for a moment, fluttering, as if unsure of where next to go, and then, as if having made a decision, landed on Mark's knee and clung there.

Fascinated by this show, Mark felt that something was being communicated to him. As he watched the butterfly's delicate wings slowly opening and closing, he felt a sense of being very close to nature. The butterfly on his leg seemed to be part of him, or he part of the butterfly, he wasn't sure which. And it wasn't just the butterfly he felt connected to—it was also the spider web, the dragonfly, and the water rippling past him as it had thirty years before.

He realized that everything around him was in balance—the butterfly with its spread wings balanced on its tiny legs; the delicate yet strong web balanced between blades of grass; and even the water, in dynamic equilibrium as it flowed between its banks. It occurred to him that a great, benevolent intelligence had been at work designing these natural objects. And since he was part of it all, then that same intelligence had designed him as well.

With that thought, he pulled a pack of cigarettes from his pocket. As he started to light one, something his doctor had said shot through his mind: "You're going to kill yourself with those." A picture flashed before his mind of his lungs having to absorb the tiny particles embedded in the smoke. He saw their natural pink color, already dark, turning even blacker. "What am I doing?" he said aloud. "God or whoever or whatever is up there created me perfectly in balance and meant for me to stay that way, in tune with nature. And when I was a kid, I was in tune. And now look at me, dirtying up my body as if I have another one in the closet that I can take out and use."

He put the cigarettes away and sat contemplating his sense of being connected to a benign universe that he had turned his back on for years. He thought hard about how he had thrown his body far out of balance—the smoke and fatty foods causing his arteries to narrow and become choked with plaque, the alcohol making his liver work overtime, the lack of exercise and extra weight placing an extra burden on his heart. He thought about how for years he had worked against the natural world surrounding him, allowing himself to be seduced by harmful substances and paying little attention to the healthful bounty that nature could provide. After an hour, the butterfly long gone, he rose and returned to his car.

Once back home, Mark used his epiphany by the stream to power his battle to kick cigarettes and alcohol, to eat better, and to exercise. Though it took effort, he made steady progress in creating a healthier lifestyle. It became easier when he found that his new regimen helped him to sleep better and to feel more energetic, less stressed out, and mentally sharper. What also helped immensely was his decision to get out into nature as much as possible. On Saturdays and Sundays, you could see Mark strolling along a nearby greenbelt or hiking the hills outside the city, taking in the natural world and feeling deeply connected to it. The psychological and social effects of Mark's decision to create a new lifestyle were as dramatic as the physical results. Almost at once, his longstanding dreary outlook began transforming into a positive engagement not only with the natural world, but with his work. His social life also picked up as he joined first a hiking group, then a birding club, making several new friends in both.

Today, Mark has blossomed into a person who is more similar to the child he used to be than to the man who allowed his body to deteriorate for years. He has stopped doing destructive things that go against his inner nature and has replaced them with healthy choices that have the blessing of outer nature. What powered this turnaround was his spiritual awakening, which led him to view the idea of healthy living in a much larger context than before. Previously his frame of reference had been constructed mostly of shoulds: "I should eat better; I should exercise; my doctor says I should quit smoking . . ." And as often happens with "shoulds," although they were true, they failed to motivate Mark to a healthier lifestyle. His epiphany was to start seeing himself as an integral part of a benevolent and intelligent universe that gives birth to life and designs organisms to be balanced and healthy. Based on this fundamentally spiritual way of viewing himself and his health, Mark realized that his previous behaviors were not only contrary to his own nature, but contrary to nature itself.

The simple yet profound ideas that changed Mark's life are at the heart of Ayurveda, which holds that our inherent state is to be in harmony with nature. We are born in balance, each one of us miraculous in our physical complexity, ability to think, capacity to care, and ability to reach spiritual depth. And though we live in a double-edged universe, nature has given us the means to stay in balance. We do so by partaking of its beneficial gifts and avoiding what we know is harmful. Doing so is only natural, because the life force is strong in each of us. We can feel it in our will to live and to grow. In this way, too, we are in harmony with nature, because the universe itself means for us to grow and flourish.

Like Mark before his transformation, many of us have no broad context in terms of which to think about health and wellness. In an age where artificial environments are the norm, it is easy to forget that we are part of nature. In a world where immediate gratification determines too many actions, it is easy to convince ourselves that it is all right to partake of temptations even if we know they are harming us. But the deep truth is that we remain nature's children through and through. Illness is a matter of losing our equilibrium in relation to the natural world. Wellness is a matter of balancing our inner constitution—physical, mental, social, and spiritual—with nature's many gifts and demands.

This Ayurvedic outlook is as pertinent today as it was five thousand years ago, and I urge you to ponder how it applies to your own health. I hope you will take a hint from Mark's story and contemplate the profound idea that Spirit—no matter how you conceive it, whether as a personal God, Brahman, or in some other way—infuses the world. When you go out into nature, realize that you are part of all you see, as natural as the birds, the trees, and the clouds. And like them, you are meant to live your life in balance with the natural world in all dimensions of your being.

EXERCISES FOR PRINCIPLE 1: AYURVEDA

Exercise 1: *Understanding Your Personal Constitution*

Your *Prakriti* is your basic constitution, which can be described in terms of three bio-energetic forces called *doshas*:

Vata – air and space

Pitta – fire and water

Kapha – water and earth

According to Ayurveda you were born with all three doshas mixed into a unique combination, but one or two of the doshas are often prevalent for an individual. There are seven possibilities: it may be that only one—Vata, Pitta, or Kapha—is prevalent; or that two—Vata-Pitta, Vata-Kapha, or Pitta Kapha—are prevalent; or that all three are present in equal measure.

To get a full and accurate evaluation of your Prakriti, you should seek out a trained and knowledgeable Ayurvedic practitioner. However, answering the questions beginning on the following page can provide you with an initial idea of which dosha or doshas are predominant for you. For each item, circle the letter or letters that you feel best describes you. Descriptions following the letter "A" correspond to Vata, those following letter "B" correspond to Pitta, and descriptions following letter "C" correspond to the Kapha dosha. When you are finished, add up the number of times you have put a circle around each letter—A, B, and C—and this will give you a rough idea of the proportion of each dosha that goes to make up your unique constitution, your Prakriti.

1. Build
   A. Small frame, usually thin, prominent joints, tendency to not easily put on weight
   B. Medium build, possibly muscular
   C. Large frame, tendency to be overweight

2. Skin
   A. Dry, rough, cool, chaps easily
   B. Oily, warm, sensitive, reddish or fair
   C. Cool, thick skin, prone to acne

3. Hair
    A. Coarse and dry, curly or frizzy
    B. Fine hair, may have balding or premature graying
    C. Thick hair, wavy, oily

4. Eyes
    A. Small, active, dark eyes
    B. Penetrating eyes, light color
    C. Large, friendly eyes

5. Lips
    A. Thin, dry, chap easily
    B. Soft, medium-sized
    C. Large, full, and smooth

6. Fingernails
    A. Brittle, ridged, or cracked
    B. Soft, flexible
    C. Thick, strong

7. Strength
    A. Little strength
    B. Moderate strength
    C. Strong with good endurance

8. Appetite
    A. Variable appetite
    B. Good appetite, tend to be irritable when hungry
    C. Strong appetite, may overeat

9. Digestion and elimination
    A. Irregular, tendency to have gas
    B. Good digestion, regular to fast evacuation
    C. Slow digestion and bowel movements

10. Amount of activity
     A. Very physically active
     B. Active, like to compete physically, well-paced activities
     C. Good stamina but less active, sometimes lethargic

11. Sleep
     A. Light sleeper, erratic
     B. Sleep well, soundly
     C. Heavy sleeper

12. Cognitive tendencies
     A. Active, creative, talkative, good recent memory, poor long-term memory
     B. Focused, aggressive, sharp, excellent memory
     C. Calm, slow, good long-term memory

13. Dominant positive emotions
     A. Cheerful, adaptive, changeable
     B. Determined, clearheaded, practical, enjoy a challenge, assertive
     C. Calm, patient, serious, compassionate but prone to attachment

14. Dominant emotions in the face of stress
     A. Tend to feel fearful, insecure, and anxious when stressed
     B. Tend to feel frustrated, irritable, impatient when stressed
     C. Tend to withdraw, avoid the situation when stressed

15. Preferred climate and other characteristics
     A. Cold hands and feet, little perspiration, do not tolerate cold well
     B. Good circulation, perspire frequently, like cold food and drinks, prefer a cool, dry climate
     C. Tendency toward respiratory congestion, tiredness, uncomfortable in cool, damp weather

Your Totals

A. _____ Vata

B. _____ Pitta

C. _____ Kapha

Below is a brief interpretation of what it means when you find that your constitution predominantly reflects one of the three doshas. If two or three of the doshas are equally prevalent for you, then according to Ayurveda your constitution is an approximately equal mixture of those two or three doshas.

People who are primarily **Vata** are generally slender and small-boned. They are cheerful, adaptable, sensitive, and enthusiastic. They like novelty and excitement, and tend to be agile both physically and in their thinking. However, vata people may be unfocused and prone to spread themselves too thinly over too many activities. Their energy level may vary, and they may lack the staying power to follow a difficult project to its completion. When stressed, they are prone to anxiety.

People who are primarily **Pitta** generally have a moderate frame, although they may be muscular and athletic. They tend to be intense, determined, focused, and intelligent. They are also ambitious and goal oriented. They are organized and attack goals and problems with a logical, one-step-at-a-time approach. Stress tends to make them frustrated and irritable.

People who are primarily **Kapha** generally have a large frame, considerable strength, and a tendency to be overweight. They are prone to be caring and compassionate and are calm and patient in temperament. Others may view them as being somewhat slow and plodding in their efforts to fulfill a goal, but they tend to be consistent in those efforts and possess a good deal of stamina. They are prone to be caring individuals, often choosing lives of service. When stressed, they tend to withdraw and avoid the stressor.

Exercise 2: *Three Crucial Areas of Balancing Inner Nature with Outer Nature*

Perhaps the main lesson we learn from Ayurveda is that physical health is a matter of balancing our inner biological nature with outer nature. This requires making sure that what we take in from outside agrees with our inner nature, that it does not harm us but instead nurtures and empowers us.

These key ideas lead to another self-evaluation exercise, one with a twofold objective. The first objective is to get you thinking about some main areas where your inner and outer nature may be either in balance or out of balance. The second is to encourage you to take action to restore the proper balance between inner and outer nature in any area where that balance is threatened.

Here are three areas where finding the proper balance between inner and outer nature is crucial for your overall wellness. Your task is to evaluate where you stand with regard to each one and then take action where necessary.

Air

Minute by minute, the single most important substance we take into our body from outside is air. We can go for days, weeks, in some cases even months without food; and we can go for hours or maybe even a day or two without water; but we can only last for a few minutes without air.

Our biological systems evolved to work best with pure, clean air. The problem is that the air most of us breathe is far from pure. Industrial discharges, vehicle emissions, cigarette smoke, household mold, and hundreds of other pollutants load the air with microscopic substances that poison our systems. To balance inner with outer nature in this area requires cleaning up and detoxifying the air you breathe. Here are two ways to help do that.

Activity: If you believe your household air is lacking in purity and healthfulness, set up one or more effective air purifiers in your home. These can help ensure that most air pollutants are scrubbed from your household air before you breathe it. Other benefits include a more restful sleep, reducing allergens in the air, and a sweeter smelling environment.

Activity: If you live in or near a city or any other major source of pollutants, take every opportunity you can to get away from airborne waste chemicals and out into nature. Go to the beach or the mountains where you can give your lungs a breathe-easier vacation. Learn how to access timely information from your local air quality board, the weather service, or other source about the concentration and movement of air pollutants in your area. Sometimes traveling only a few miles in the right direction from the city can bring you to an area with much purer, healthier air.

Water

The water we drink may be the second most important substance we take into our body from the outside. The pollutant situation is generally not nearly as serious with water as it is with air. Most municipalities and water districts do a good job of treating water for our homes. Nevertheless, there are sometimes trace chemicals in treated water that reduce its purity and healthfulness. Also, household circumstances such as eroding pipes and sediment in hot water tanks may diminish the quality of your water supply.

Activity: Evaluate the quality of your own household drinking water. If you find it lacking, then invest in a water purification system if you have not done so already. If money is an issue, several relatively inexpensive systems are available, either faucet-mounted heads or purification pitchers. As long as you replace filters according to schedule, these simple water purifiers can last for years. Additional benefits include tastier water for you and your family and the knowledge that your inner nature is thanking you with every glass of purified water you drink.

Food

The fact that you have probably many times heard the saying "You are what you eat" is testimony to the profound truth of this old homily. Ayurvedic medicine recognized that truth thousands of years ago. Almost all of us have some understanding of how a healthy diet promotes wellness and a long life; but unfortunately, most of us have too little understanding to make the best food choices to promote wellness of body. That's the purpose of this activity—to encourage you to learn more if your nutritional wisdom happens to be a little on the light side.

Activity: Locate some trustworthy sources of nutritional information, such as books, websites, or other guidelines, and learn enough to be able to address the questions on the next page. If, after answering the questions, you find one or more areas for which your actual practice differs from recommended practice, consider taking action to rectify the imbalance.

- What is the recommended number of calories per day for someone of your gender, age, activity level, and ideal weight? _____ What is your actual average number of daily calories? _____

- How do micronutrients promote wellness? _____ _____ Which micronutrients do you often have in your diet? _____

- What are three of the best sources of micronutrients that are also readily available in food stores? _____ _____

- What daily balance of fats, carbohydrates, and protein do qualified nutritionists recommend? _____ What is your average daily balance? _____

- How much salt is too much salt? _____ How much salt do you ingest each day on average? _____ What are the risk factors for ingesting too much salt? _____ _____

- How many daily servings of fresh fruit and vegetables do nutritionists recommend? _____ How many daily servings do you have? _____

PRINCIPLE 2

ℂℨ

Calmness

Quiet the Turbulence

"If thou art pained by any external thing, it is not the thing
that disturbs you, but your own judgment about it. And
it is in your power to wipe out this judgment now."

Marcus Aurelius
from *Meditations,* Book VII

Stress has been called the ailment of our time, with up to seventy percent of doctor visits being related to stress. This is not surprising in a fast-paced world where potentially stressful situations may face us at every turn. The demands of work, finances, relationships, and other issues can seem unending. Some people are able to handle those demands better than others. But for many, such pressures create the ongoing mental, emotional, physiological, and spiritual turbulence that characterizes chronic stress.

It's not that all stress is bad. Suppose that on your lunch break you walk around a corner and find yourself confronted by an African lion. Right away, you experience a state of acute psychological stress: *It's a lion! And it's right there in front of me!* Your physiology immediately responds to what your eyes are telling you. A host of hormones rush into your blood, readying your body for action. Your senses become super sharp. Your cells pump out extra energy. Your breathing rate increases to provide you more oxygen. Your heart pumps faster so your blood can quickly move the extra energy to your muscles.

This reaction, called *the stress response,* begins within a second or two of your initial perception. It has evolved as a necessary physiological device to help quickly prepare someone—in this case, you—to confront a potentially dangerous situation. It is also called the *fight or flight response.* You can either stand your ground and fight the lion, or you can take flight, perhaps by running inside a building or climbing a telephone pole. That's

19

what your stress response is preparing you to do: one or the other. But once the danger has passed—once you realize the lion lurking there on the sidewalk is actually a realistic-looking, life-sized stuffed animal displayed outside a high-end toy store—your body quickly returns to its normal state. The hormones stop pouring out, your heart slows, your breathing returns to its regular rate, and all your other bodily systems resume their usual activities. And now you'll have a good story to tell on yourself when you get back to work.

We can be thankful that this acute version of stress takes over our physiology when we are confronted by an outside physical threat. The same sort of reaction may also kick into gear and tune us up at times when we need to give our best performance, such as in presenting a speech or driving on an icy road. But unfortunately, there is another version of stress, one that involves repeated psychologically taxing events over a substantial period of time. This is chronic stress, and it can arise from many sources—difficult life situations such as marital problems, working at a job that makes us unhappy, the day-to-day pressures of living, and much more.

The Ugly Legacy of Chronic Stress

What makes the chronic version of stress so problematic is that the same physiological reactions occur as with acute stress; but because the turbulence is ongoing, our body doesn't return to its normal state. The extra hormones continue circulating in our blood, unbalancing and gradually damaging bodily systems. Research shows that chronic stress promotes cardiovascular disease, diabetes, immune system deterioration, and a host of other ailments. Over time, this can add up to major physical problems. In the final analysis, chronic stress is a potential killer.

And it's not only our physical health that is put at risk by repeated stress. Ongoing turbulence also seriously detracts from our emotional and social well-being. This is because stress causes deep as opposed to shallow turbulence. Shallow turbulence can be represented by a squall out on the ocean. Inside the squall, a great commotion is taking place. The rain is pouring down in buckets while a powerful, swirling wind churns the ocean's surface into a choppy mess. But ten yards below, the water is calm. Fish, octopi, and dolphins go on their peaceful ways undisturbed by the tempest lashing the waves into a foaming maelstrom directly above. The turbulence goes only a few feet down. Its force is quickly dampened and absorbed by the water below.

It's a different story for deep turbulence. Here too, the action begins with some disturbance at the surface. But the agitation quickly travels to other parts of the system, creating tumultuous and unbalanced conditions everywhere. That's what happens with chronic stress. The discord starts at the surface of our mind with a perception, experience, or idea that causes anxiety or trepidation. Almost instantaneously it transmits itself to deeper parts of our biological and mental structure. In a few blinks of an eye, it has gone all the way down, creating turbulence throughout our bodily systems, profoundly affecting not only our physiology, but also our thoughts, emotions, behaviors, and attitudes.

Stress can also have many indirect impacts. It can prevent us from getting the precious sleep we need to stay healthy and at our best. Instead, we lie in bed wide awake, thoughts racing a mile a minute as we play and replay scenarios related to whatever is preying on our mind. Stress is also a main cause for addictive behaviors such as overeating and alcohol abuse, which can create physiological harm as devastating as the runaway hormones. The combination of direct and indirect physiological impacts makes stress into a double whammy pounding away at our physical health.

Chronic stress also affects the way we get along with family, friends, and others, detracting from our quality of life. Instead of enjoying the movie with our friend or partner, we sit there in a blur, worrying how we'll make the next mortgage payment. At the office picnic we may act like we're having fun, but as we make half-hearted conversation, that difficult issue we've been having with the neighbors or the boss is simmering in the back of our mind. Ironically, when under stress, we sometimes push away family members and friends who might help us relax and forget our perceived troubles.

Mental turbulence also tends to infect other thought processes. Anxiety about one issue may lead us to worry about others. We start seeing trouble everywhere. When we experience the world this way, it becomes even harder to take our mind off what we perceive to be our troubles and find joy in life. Stress narrows our thinking and creates cognitive blind spots. It can hinder us from seeking ways to handle whatever is causing the stress. Our agitated thinking may keep us from seeing a solution right in front of our face.

Given its many harmful effects, it is abundantly clear that learning how to deal effectively with stress is of paramount importance if we are to achieve the deep, energized wellness that we desire.

Methods for Calming the Turbulence

The good news is that there are excellent strategies to calm the turbulence caused by repeated stress. The most obvious may be to *Change the Stressor*, which is the situation that leads us to feel stressed. For instance, if our job constantly drives us up the wall, one solution would be to find a job that suits us better. Or if we're anxious about contracting cardiovascular disease, a very reasonable strategy to reduce our stress would be to work with our physician to develop a heart-healthy plan, and then enact the plan.

Sometimes, though, it is difficult to change a potential stressor. If we find ourselves fuming about being caught in a traffic jam, there is usually nothing much we can do to change the external situation. We just have to wait it out. That's where a second basic strategy for dealing with stress comes in: *Reframe the Situation*. This strategy is based on the idea that although the things we get stressed about are out in the world, our way of thinking about them is in our mind. And it is our way of thinking about them that determines whether they provoke the stress response.

For example, consider something most of us have experienced—a day on which everything seems to go "wrong." When a series of minor mishaps occur, we can take a narrow or a broad view. On the narrow view, we assign the events more importance than they deserve. As they pile up, we start feeling overwhelmed and stressed out. On the broader view, we regard the events as no more than minor bumps strung out along our path. We take them in stride, perhaps laughing at our "bad luck" on this particular day. For the most part, we stay calm and stress free. The difference is our attitude. If people would always take the broader perspective when faced with potential stressors, much of the chronic stress that permeates our society would disappear.

There are many ways to help ourselves to take that broader view. Some are physiologically based. These include getting enough sleep and exercising regularly, both of which strengthen our ability to take a calm, philosophical approach to potential stressors. For example, after a stressful day at work, instead of collapsing in a chair to lose yourself and your troubles temporarily in the television, a wiser course would be to go for a leisurely walk in a nearby park, perhaps with your spouse, significant other, or friend. Certainly, getting absorbed in mindless entertainment may temporarily alleviate stress, but when the TV shows are over, the thought processes that led to the stress may return in full force. On the other hand, while taking a pleasant walk, the physical exercise alone tends to calm down the worried mind and create space for new perspectives that could serve to reduce the stressful feelings.

Other strategies involve our social dimension—Heart. Usually, an effective way to deal with persistent stress is to talk about your feelings with someone, a friend or relative, who cares about your well-being. Unfortunately, many people are hesitant to do this for one reason or another. It may be that they are reluctant to "lay their troubles" on someone else. This stoic attitude may be especially prevalent among men, but it is also a feature of many women's personalities. Such individuals may think they should shoulder any perceived trouble solely by themselves, thinking that not to do so would indicate some kind of character flaw. Others may have had unpleasant experiences in sharing with others, feeling they did not find the understanding and caring ear they hoped for. Yet others may simply feel embarrassed to share their perceptions even with friends because of the nature of the trouble, e.g., marital or other family-related issues that they feel must remain private.

However, none of these rationales constitute a good enough reason not to share our perceived stressful burdens by talking about them with someone we trust. It is not a character flaw to tell caring others how we feel about some problem we may be having. And we need not expect the future to necessarily be the same as the past, even if we have been disappointed in the past by the quality of someone's listening. Even for private issues that cause stress, we can always find someone appropriate to talk to—if not a family member or good friend, then a trusted pastor or counselor.

The bottom line is that to share our perceptions, disappointments, and worries with others is almost always helpful for alleviating stress. Even just to joke with a friend at lunch about our "troubles," whatever they may be, can be therapeutic. The laughter helps put them in perspective and reduce stressful feelings

Reframing Ourselves Spiritually

Our most powerful strategy for defusing stress by reframing the stressful situation arises out of our fourth dimension of being—Spirit. Because this dimension is about looking at what happens in our lives from a wide, all-encompassing viewpoint, it is perfectly suited for providing the broad perspectives that counteract stress. This is true no matter what our spiritual beliefs may be. For example, countless people find their anxieties greatly assuaged by belief in a fatherly God who has their best interests in mind. Others, of a different spiritual persuasion, may view their relationship with a Higher Reality as being like that of a wave to an ocean. Their sense that they are part of something much larger than themselves is a calming influence. Still others may find that their contemplation of perennial values such as Truth, Love, Family, Beauty, or Art helps provide the larger perspective that makes potential stressors lose their bite.

One basic reason chronic stress is rampant in our society is that so many people have allowed their spiritual dimension to atrophy. Without powerful and enduring spiritual beliefs, we have no larger context in terms of which to view what happens in our lives. When we lack that larger context, events are defined only by whether they promote or hinder the achievement of whatever objectives we are currently pursuing. And these are almost always ego-centered when Spirit is absent. As a result, when a potentially stressful event pops up, it appears to us as a hated enemy threatening our progress. It is difficult to see it in any other way. The result is the stress response, often repeated dozens of times a day.

But we can turn this around. By cultivating our spiritual dimension, we can develop effective tools that enable us to reframe the "mishaps," large and small, that occur in all of our lives, enabling us to escape the destructive grip of stress. These tools consist of spiritually based principles and truths that enable us to see our lives in terms of broader, more enlightened perspectives. The principles and truths presented in this book can help defuse potentially stressful events.

We have learned about Emily, who was faced with a lot of job-related stress caused by her having assumed new responsibilities. The continued stress was hurting her physiologically, psychologically, and socially—that is, in Body, Mind, and Heart. She started questioning her purpose in life and the value of her work. What began making a difference in Emily's life was meditation (something we will learn more about below). Meditating enabled Emily to create mental space to re-evaluate her priorities and see more clearly what was most important in her life. She realized that what was most meaningful to her was her family, doing a good job at her work, and the joys and satisfactions that came from embracing these two main aspects of her experience. These are spiritual perspectives because they constituted for Emily a broad, all-encompassing view of the significance of her life.

Why couldn't Emily have realized these things to begin with? This is because one of the destructive results of chronic stress is that it narrows our vision and over-emphasizes the seriousness of whatever situation gives rise to the stress, often making it seem worse than it actually is. Meditation helped Emily break through the incessant repetition of thought processes that typically accompany and exacerbate chronic stress. We don't know exactly what thought processes these were for Emily. Perhaps she saw herself as unable to perform her new responsibilities well enough. Maybe she was afraid of being unable to balance her work with her family life. There are any number of stories Emily could have told herself that nagged her and produced stress.

But meditation gave her the space to start breaking through these thought processes and gain some new perspectives. By embracing her spiritual dimension and reflecting on what gave her most meaning in life, Emily reframed her situation in broad strokes. She took a dark drawing in charcoal, which was her stress-saturated view of her situation, and painted it over with new, brighter, more colorful strokes. In doing so, she did not change anything that was actually present *in* her situation; she simply saw it in a new perspective. As we will see repeatedly in future chapters, this is how contemplating basic spiritual principles can effectively change our perceptions of ourselves and the world. If our old perceptions and ways of engaging with the world were leading to chronic stress, our new viewpoint, being more in tune with Spirit, helps defuse the stress.

When you accept these basic spiritual principles both cognitively and emotionally, they can make a profound difference in your life. This includes their ability to serve as an antidote to persistent stress, as Emily discovered. But if the principles are to do much more than just sit on the page, it is crucial that you understand and reflect on how they can order and empower your daily life. They must become more than theoretical,

Spiritual Principles: The Best Reframer

We all face challenges at one time or another, sometimes ones that may threaten to debilitate us. I certainly have.

A few years ago, there was a time when my stress level almost rocketed out of control because of serious health issues. This was the period I called *The Dark Night of the Soul* in the preface to this book. It occurred not long after I had begun the journey into understanding and teaching Mind-Body-Spirit medicine, and it threatened to become a huge roadblock on that journey. For a time, it seemed I was becoming weaker and weaker by the day, and my mind often played catastrophic scenarios about sickness and death that left me feeling almost hopeless. But thankfully, some of the same spiritual principles I had been learning about came to my rescue.

One of the most important of these was the Principle of Acceptance, which you will learn more about in the next chapter. Aided by meditation, my reflection on this principle helped calm my anxieties and foster a sense that ultimately, all is right with the world and with me. I learned not to fight against my condition emotionally but to accept it. This freed me to better use my intelligence and energy to deal with my situation positively and work toward the best outcome. This change in attitude also helped defuse my catastrophic thinking and its resulting stress and helped my body to heal.

Another main spiritual principle that came to my aid was Practice the Virtues of Heart, the topic of Principle 7. It came to me in the form of the love and support given me by my family, love that made me stronger in Body and all other dimensions.

Today, the health issues are gone. What remains is a deep understanding of how adhering to spiritual principles can relieve stress and foster hope and even joy in the face of trouble.

more than just another set of good ideas, more than something for you to put on the back burner and think about at some later time. If the thesis of this book is correct, you cannot afford to skim over the ideas and principles presented here. Your wellness in all dimensions of your being is intimately affected by your spiritual aspect. If you welcome the principles of Spirit into your daily life, your wellness will benefit not just in your spiritual aspect but in Body, Mind, and Heart.

Embracing Calmness through Meditation

One of the best ways to embrace calmness is through meditation, which releases the calming influence of Spirit. There are various kinds of meditation. The one I want to explain here we can call "sitting meditation." It is expressly designed to tone down your mind's chatter, calm your body, and help you create a more peaceful approach to life's ups and downs. It counteracts the stress response by promoting a *relaxation response* that restores your body's natural balance. Here is a simple procedure that can get you meditating right away.

- Choose a word or short phrase that means something to you, such as "Love" or "Life is great." This is your focus word or phrase.

- In a quiet room, assume a comfortable sitting position on a straight-backed chair or, if you prefer, cross-legged on the floor with your back straight. Make sure the room temperature is comfortable, not too warm or cool. Rest your hands comfortably in your lap.

- Now close your eyes and breathe slowly in and out through your nose. Allow the air to go deep into your diaphragm, expanding your belly, then breathe out. Slowly, slowly, in and out, taking nice deep breaths.

- As you inhale and exhale, don't think of anything, just feel the movements of your chest and diaphragm, back and forth, back and forth. Each time you exhale, repeat silently to yourself your focus word or phrase.

- Maintain an accepting attitude toward what you are doing. Don't worry whether you are doing it right. If thoughts enter your mind, say to yourself something like, "It's okay" or "Don't worry" and let the thoughts drift away. Go back to simply experiencing your breathing movements, repeating your focus item each time you exhale.

- When you feel it is time to end the session, sit quietly, eyes closed, for a minute. Let other thoughts enter your mind naturally. Then open your eyes and sit calmly for another minute before rising.

This kind of meditation can help treat a range of stress-related disorders. Daily meditation for fifteen to thirty minutes in the morning can reduce stress throughout the day. It may take time to build up to that amount, however. You may want to start by meditating for five or ten minutes and then add more time as you become more comfortable with the procedure. The first session or two you may feel yourself getting bored or dozing off. If so, don't let that stop you. Gently remind yourself that you are supposed to be focusing on your breathing and get back to doing that.

Not only can meditation reduce stress directly, it can also help create the quiet, reflective mental environment that enables you to better contemplate the spiritual ideas and principles permeating this book. To help foster this calm and receptive attitude as you read, I suggest beginning each chapter with a brief mini-meditation, as described in the following first exercise.

EXERCISES FOR PRINCIPLE 2: CALMNESS

Exercise 1: *Learn to Do Mini-Meditations*

Meditation is a wonderful way to counteract stress, and meditating for ten, fifteen, or thirty minutes at a certain time each day, say in the morning, can have salutary effects. But meditation can also be done on short notice, and for only a minute or two, perhaps even at your workplace. These are *mini-meditations,* and they too can help you relax and counteract stress.

Your exercise here is to practice mini-meditating. Mini-meditations are similar to regular meditations, which you learned about earlier in the chapter, but they take less time.

For example, if you are sitting in your office and need to reset your mind and body due to stress, begin by making yourself comfortable and, insofar as possible, blocking out extraneous noise. Then close your eyes and begin breathing in and out deeply and rhythmically.

While you do this, focus your experience on the movements of your chest and diaphragm. Feel how your chest and belly expand as you inhale and deflate as you exhale. Each time you exhale, silently say to yourself your focus word or phrase. This might be, for example, a loved person's name, or the phrase "the world is beautiful." Do this for a set number of breaths, perhaps a dozen or so, or for a minute or more. When you feel it is time, sit quietly for a moment with eyes closed. Then open your eyes and feel the refreshing sense of calmness that came from your mini-meditation. You should only have to do this a few times before it becomes a natural tool that you can use most anytime to counteract stress and calm your thought and feeling processes.

Exercise 2: *Reframe Stressful Situations*

Here is an exercise that you can perform at the moment a stressful situation appears, or later when you reflect on how you perceived the situation. The idea here is to do two things. First, understand how your perception of the situation adds to its stressful nature. Next, find one or more ways to mentally reframe the situation so that it loses its power to bring about stress. Let me illustrate these ideas with a couple of examples.

You are hard at work in your office cubicle or on the work line when you think you overhear two co-workers making a joke about some aspect of your appearance, work, or other behavior. Your body immediately goes into stress mode as a host of hormones pour out into your bloodstream and your blood pressure rises. At once you start telling yourself a story about how your co-workers are belittling you and how you will "get back" at the offenders, perhaps by confronting them. But then you recall that you are supposed to be doing this reframing exercise, in which you try to perceive the situation in a new, plausible, less stressful way. So you decide to do that.

First, you remember that you're not even sure you heard what you assume you heard. You thought you heard your name but maybe you were mistaken in that. Then you realize that even if what you heard was a reference to you, people often poke a little fun at others whom they genuinely like. You've probably done that yourself. So your interpretation of what you think you heard as somehow belittling you may be way off the mark.

Finally, you realize that it doesn't really matter in the broader context whether the co-workers were being "catty" toward you or not. They don't pay your salary, and you have friends who love and respect you. All of these thoughts can be helpful in calming your stressful feelings and getting you back focused on your work. Later, if you reflect on the incident, you can probably come up with even more interpretations that will serve to defuse it.

Another situation that might cause stress is being late for a meeting because you are caught in a traffic jam. Instead of sitting there fuming, thinking about how this means you will have to enter the meeting late, reframe the situation. One way you can do so is by realizing that the others at the meeting will most likely understand your predicament and not blame you for being late. After all, we all know about traffic jams. They're uncontrollable. They simply pop up in your life, often without warning and at the most inconvenient times. You can further reframe your situation by realizing that in the "grand scheme of things" traffic jams are just another minor hindrance that we sometimes must face. Chances are extremely high that your happening to be in one right now will have no permanent bearing on your life. But what may have a very large bearing is your learning how to rethink and reframe such situations so they don't become very stressful. Learning that lesson could help defuse a great deal of stress over time and add years to your life.

Now for the exercise proper. Consider two or three recent stressful incidents you experienced. Set down on a piece of paper or a computer screen how you interpreted each incident—what ways of thinking about the incident brought on the stress? Next, set down three ways you could have reframed each incident—three plausible things you could have told yourself at the time that would have defused the incident. Notice, as you do this exercise, how easy and even natural it is to interpret an incident that is neutral in itself as being unfavorable to you personally. We often tend to think the worst when something happens that we can view in that way. One of the values of reframing is that it teaches us that we don't have to accept our first interpretation of an incident. In this way, it expands our mind and our horizons.

PRINCIPLE 3

☙

Acceptance
Work with the River of Life

*"By letting it go it all gets done. The world is won by
those who let it go. But when you try and try,
the world is beyond the winning."*

Lao-Tzu
from *Tao Te Ching*

Life has often been described as a kind of battle. But it is not clear who or what we are supposed to be fighting against. The world? Society? Time? Death? To view life as an ongoing battle is certainly one way to look at it. But it is not a helpful viewpoint if our goal is to achieve total wellness. It is also an attitude that has been strongly challenged by the greatest religious traditions. Virtually every major religious and spiritual movement has recognized the great value of assuming an attitude of acceptance toward what happens in life. For example, both Buddhism and Hinduism champion the idea of not fighting against life but rather moving harmoniously with its flow day by day. And both Christianity and Judaism teach the wisdom, indeed the necessity, of accepting God's will in whatever occurs in our lives.

The Power of Maintaining an Attitude of Acceptance

The spiritual idea of maintaining an attitude of acceptance toward our experience is a powerful antidote to stress. Why this is so becomes clear when we realize that psychological stress is, in its essence, a kind of emotional opposition to what we experience. It begins with a perception that something is a threat to us or our goals. The stressor may be something we think has happened, is happening, or will happen. In any event, our perception that this something is a threat triggers an emotional response in opposition to it. This emotional opposition appears in the form of worry, anxiety, fear, or other psychological distress. The stronger our emotional resistance to the perceived threat, the stronger our stress response.

But suppose that instead of emotionally opposing a potential stressor, we accepted it. Suppose that we reasoned that if some event occurs, then there is no getting around it—it occurs. So why emotionally resist it? Why rail against it? Opposing it emotionally won't make it go away. It will only result in psychological distress and hormones running rampant through our body. It's reality—so why not accept it?

This attitude of not opposing reality is a reflection of one of the most profound of all spiritual principles, the Principle of Acceptance:

> *Do not set yourself against reality emotionally but accept it as it is.*
> *Then employ this acceptance to empower you*
> *to become your fullest self.*

By assuming the attitude toward our experience that this principle advocates, we avoid the emotional resistance to reality on which chronic stress relies. By accepting the situations and circumstances reality brings to us, stress has no opportunity to arise.

When I advocate the Principle of Acceptance, people sometimes misunderstand. They think I am talking about being passive, resigned, and apathetic about whatever may happen to us. But that is not it at all. The Principle of Acceptance entails a very positive and active approach to life. In fact, embracing the principle wholeheartedly does much more than alleviate stress. It is one of our most powerful tools for creating our lives according to our dreams and aspirations.

This is easier to see if we first understand that we cannot possibly win by opposing reality. To fail to accept our experience is to fight a losing battle because nothing exists but reality. And to deny reality is to affirm nothing. On the other hand, by emotionally accepting what we experience in our lives, we necessarily align ourselves with reality—with all that is. And because reality is infused with Spirit (a lesson you will find repeated again and again in this book) we align ourselves with Spirit when we align with reality.

Does that mean we must acquiesce to whatever conditions or situations we come across in our experience? Does it mean we must always accept reality as we find it and never try to change a state of affairs to what we consider to be a better or more hopeful condition? No. It simply means that we must give up flailing against the situation emotionally. For example, if we are considering a circumstance where someone is treating someone else unjustly, it will do little good to get angry and stomp around at the injustice of it all. A much more effective approach would be to calm down emotionally, realize that this is the way things are at the moment, and accept that reality. Then, with our eyes and mind clearer because of the absence of anger and angst, we can muster a calm determination and start exploring the ways in which we might change the situation so the injustice is alleviated. In this way, emotional acceptance of the reality in front of us does not lead to acquiescence. On the contrary, it helps empower us by clearing our head so we can better devise methods to effect the change we believe is needed.

The popular media often show the Principle of Acceptance at work, where it is portrayed as a precondition for overcoming some challenge. For example, you have probably read or seen dozens of stories and movies of people who face a difficult disability or other problem and who begin by thrashing around emotionally for a time. Then gradually, they begin accepting their situation. That's the point where their mind clears and they can begin the process of overcoming the challenge through their efforts. Part of the moral of such stories is that opposing reality emotionally simply does not work. A necessary condition to bring about change is to stop fighting what is. All of these stories show the Principle of Acceptance at work and give a lesson for our lives. Whatever potentially stressful situations we may encounter in our experience, whether they are about relationships, work, finances, health, or something else, acceptance of the reality confronting us is the first step to calming the turbulence inside and dealing effectively with the situation.

To not resist the reality we encounter is also a main principle found in the martial arts. For example, in learning judo, one is taught not to resist the opponent directly but to accept the opponent's movements and leverage them for our own purposes. Our intention in applying judo is certainly to defend ourselves and defeat the opponent, but acceptance rather than resistance is the key strategy. Similarly, in other areas of life, accepting rather than resisting a reality that seems to stand in our way helps to empower our efforts to deal with that reality.

The River of Life

To grasp these ideas better, we can use the metaphor of the River of Life in which we think of life as a river that you are floating and swimming down. Sometimes the river flows slowly and sometimes swiftly, bending this way and that as different situations arise. Other people in your life, your family, friends, and others, are accompanying you on the River of Life. At any point one or more of them may be near you, while others may be on some other part of the river.

Let us suppose that someone on the river, a friend of yours, is approaching an event that will occur in a few days downstream. This is a meeting with her banker about being behind in her mortgage payments. The prospect of this meeting seems threatening to your friend. She sees no good coming from it. Dreading the event, she starts to feel like it is a big jagged rock in the middle of the river. What will happen when she hits the rock? She imagines that foreclosure will quickly follow. She starts desperately trying to think of some way to avoid the rock. She uses all her mental energy stressing out about it, wanting to swim away from it, wanting to be in some other situation. In effect, she is trying, at least mentally, to swim against the river, to deny the reality she is approaching. But she seems unable to do so. The river is too powerful. All she does is flail around, making a lot of useless waves while the river takes her closer and closer to the "big jagged rock."

Now let us say that you, too, are approaching a similar situation on the River of Life and that the same considerations that seem to threaten your friend are present in your own meeting. That is, you are going to meet with your banker to discuss the mortgage you are two months behind on. Unlike your friend, however, you have fully accepted that the meeting will occur. You are not in a state of emotional opposition. The meeting does not feel to you like a big rock that you are about to crash into. Certainly, you might prefer to be doing something else that day, but you are not in a state of denial. And you acknowledge the possibility that the meeting will end with the bank representative deciding to initiate foreclosure proceedings. But you have accepted all that. You have played through this scenario in your mind. At first, the prospect of foreclosure seemed to you as if it would be a catastrophe for you and your family. But after some anxious moments you came to realize that if this scenario were actually to develop, you and your family would land on your feet. You would have learned some lessons, and new opportunities would eventually open up.

As a result, you not wasting your mental, emotional, and physical energies fretting about the situation. Instead, you are using those energies to prepare for the meeting. You realize that the opportunity for a frank discussion could give you your best chance to save your house, possibly through refinancing. Instead of wasting your mental energy by flailing around on the River of Life, you are moving calmly toward the upcoming situation, using your substantial brain power to figure out the best way to approach it. In fact, you feel yourself swimming *toward* the event. You accept that it is in your future, but not passively. You are approaching the meeting with a plan in mind, taking some sure, deft strokes that should help you deal effectively with it. The thing that enables you to take those sure strokes instead of wasting your energy flailing around is your attitude of acceptance. And far from making you passive or resigned, this attitude allows you to approach the meeting calmly, effectively, and positively.

Are you and your friend on the same river? Yes. But what a difference! Facing the same kind of situation, the two of you perceive two different realities. Why does your attitude differ from your friend's? Perhaps it's because you have reflected more on the ups and downs of life. You have come to understand that by assuming an attitude of acceptance, you are able to take advantage of the River's enormous power to energize your swimming as you move through life. You know that when you give up your worries and anxieties, it's like giving up a leaden belt weighing you down. And when you emotionally accept what is given to you in your experience, it's like putting on a pair of big, new swim fins. They enable you to swim farther and faster, with renewed power and grace, as you take steps to deal with whatever situations arise.

And that's exactly what you are doing in this case. While your friend flounders and flails, emotionally opposing what is coming, you have accepted its reality and are swimming directly toward it. As you do so, you develop a plan that will give you your very best chance of coming out of the meeting with a result you want. It doesn't guarantee your success, but it makes success much more likely.

But what if, despite your best efforts, the results of the meeting are not to your liking? What if that foreclosure scenario you entertained for a short time actually develops? Should you continue to assume an attitude

The Principle of Acceptance Leads to the Beautiful Water

The Principle of Acceptance has entered my life in many ways, including opening up new experiences that I otherwise would have missed. Let me give you an example.

One of my sons was in medical school, and I was visiting him for several days. On this particular afternoon he was in class, and I was walking along a beach near my apartment. It was a sunny day, and the clear blue water of the ocean beckoned me. But I had brought no swimsuit on my trip, so I merely stood there longing to be in the surf. After a moment the thought came that I could remove my shoes and wade into the water pants, shirt, and all. But there were strangers around me on the beach and in the water, and I felt they would think me odd. So I continued to stand there, longing to be in the inviting water.

Then a question struck me: What did it matter what others thought if I went in clothes still on? Sure, some might think me odd. But so what? I could live with that reality. With that thought, I laid my wallet, keys, and belt on my overshirt, removed my shoes and socks, and splashed myself right into the azure water. It was glorious. I walked out a little way, sat down waist deep, and felt the warm sun and a soft breeze caressing my head. I stayed there for almost half an hour, playing and enjoying the ocean, feeling Spirit all around and within me. Then I got out and walked barefoot to my apartment dripping pure, clean water all the way.

This was the Principle of Acceptance at work in my life. I could have let my concern for others' opinions dictate my afternoon. Instead, I fully accepted the reality that some people might not approve of my splashing in the surf with my clothes on. If they do, they do, I thought—no matter. It was that acceptance of imagined reality that led me to then go jump into and experience that beautiful beckoning ocean.

of acceptance? Yes, yes, yes! Whatever happens at the meeting will be your new reality. It must be accepted and dealt with. But you already know that. You've already accepted that possibility. And you know you do not have time to waste your emotional energies feeling sorry for yourself or flailing around like your friend did. Of course you hope the meeting goes well for you. That's what all the planning has been for. But whatever happens at the meeting, you will accept it and then use your best thinking and planning to determine how best to proceed.

Accepting Others

A special aspect of following the Principle of Acceptance is to apply it to the people we encounter in our lives. We do this by not opposing them emotionally but rather accepting them for who they are.

We humans have a tendency to negatively evaluate other people and groups of people who we feel are sufficiently unlike us or who seem somehow to threaten us by their very existence. This characteristic may have served a survival function at one time because of the necessity for prehistoric humans to band together in groups for safety. But if so, it is a characteristic that has long outlived its usefulness. Yet it continues largely unabated in the world today. People still find it easy to develop a degree of emotional negativity toward others who do not adhere to their concept of what a person should be or believe. This fact is brought home to us virtually every day as we witness racial, ethnic, religious, and nationalistic prejudices on a broad scale. For many, it is also evident in their daily lives as they find themselves emotionally opposed to individuals that they judge as being too this or too that: lazy or too ambitious, arrogant or a doormat, a cold fish or too friendly, slovenly or a neat freak. These and thousands of other negative categorizations of others are applied countless times every day. The felt antagonism toward the guy who lives across the street or works down the hall may not be voiced directly to his face, but the negative judgments are there, unspoken, along with their emotional baggage.

If we take a broad view of all this activity, it is immediately clear that the negativity present in these judgments is actually not a feature of the other person, but of the judgment itself. Whether we judge a woman as arrogant or a doormat, whether we judge a man as slovenly or a neat freak, the people we are judging are just who they are. The concepts *arrogant, doormat, slovenly,* and *neat freak* are not categories invented by God, Brahman, Buddha, or Nature. They were invented by humans for human purposes, and the main human purpose they serve is to categorize people negatively. The problem is that by applying such categories to the people we meet, we obstruct our ability to recognize their complex, rich humanity. If we categorize someone that we know as being lazy, a cold fish, or unfriendly, this is who they become for us—that and nothing else. Innumerable aspects of their reality are obliterated in our mind, an enormous loss both to those who are judged and those who do the judging.

To avoid this loss, it is crucial to apply the Principle of Acceptance in our dealings with others, to accept, not oppose, the reality of the other person in all of its richness. To do so is to refuse to categorize others in terms of concepts that pack a negative emotional wallop. It is to approach others with good will and an open mind, acknowledging their personhood. This does not require that we be naive about the people we meet. We can approach new acquaintances positively and still be wary, understanding that there are those in the world who would take advantage of us. Of course, the fact is that most humans are decent and moral people who dream, work hard, and seek fulfillment just as we do. And this is true no matter what their race, ethnicity, religion, nationality, gender, age, occupation, party, education, or personal style. To refuse to jump to a negative conclusion about someone based on their behavior, beliefs, or any other fact about them, to accept them as we find them in all their beautiful and complex reality, is a blessed way of relating to our fellow humans.

Jason's Liberation from His Attitude toward a Client

To recognize that our judgments of others are ultimately labels that we ourselves produce and must take responsibility for can be liberating. This is illustrated by an incident that happened to a young man I'll call Jason.

Jason worked as a self-employed financial advisor in a one-man office. Among his twenty or so clients was a man named Chuck, whose personality Jason could barely tolerate. Chuck had several particular behaviors that irritated Jason. For example, every time Chuck entered Jason's office, he made what Jason interpreted as a snide comment. He would say that the office furniture looked old, mention that Jason needed a haircut, or point out some other perceived fault. After the first few meetings, Jason began to dislike Chuck so much that he could barely eke out a welcoming smile for him when he came through the door. He contemplated dropping Chuck, but he couldn't afford losing a client, so he decided he would just have to put up with the man. This he did, though he would always become very stiff and formal when Chuck arrived, secretly thinking him an arrogant fool.

One day Chuck came into the office with Amy, his wife of ten years, to discuss their financial affairs. Jason found Amy to be pleasant, pretty, and intelligent, and she had obvious affection for Chuck. Somewhat surprised, Jason realized that Amy obviously didn't see Chuck as an arrogant fool.

One night soon after, Jason came across an Internet business article about dealing with others. It included a statement that struck Jason as curious: "If there's a fool out there, you created him." This seemed so obviously false to Jason, that he muttered, "That's ridiculous." But as he read the statement's rationale, he began to understand that the writer was only saying that someone who labels someone else with the negative concept "fool" is making a choice. The "fool" likely has friends who do not apply that category. For them, the person is not a fool. He or she may exhibit behaviors that might lead some people to apply the word "fool," but other people see those behaviors in a different light and do not apply that word.

Jason thought of Chuck and his judgment that Chuck was an arrogant fool. Was the article right? Was Jason the one who was creating Chuck as a fool? He remembered Chuck's wife Amy. Evidently, she didn't create Chuck as a fool. Then the idea that he was the one responsible for labeling Chuck with the concept arrogant fool struck him full force. That's exactly right, he thought, Chuck is a fool for me only insofar as I think of him that way. But I don't have to do that. Maybe some of his behaviors irritate me, but I don't have to let that fact govern my way of categorizing him or engaging with him.

Suddenly, Jason was infused with a sense of liberation and power. He recalled that it was almost painful to smile at Chuck when he entered the office, and he realized that his inability to smile was because he thought of Chuck so negatively. But he didn't have to do that. He didn't have to like Chuck, but he also didn't have to dislike him. He could just let Chuck be Chuck. Jason wondered, "Can I actually do that"? Then he realized that tomorrow would be a good test. Chuck was scheduled to come by in the morning for a short discussion. And that meeting would be a good test for whether Jason's attitude toward Chuck was really changed.

Sure enough, at ten the next morning, Chuck entered Jason's office. His first words were, "You need more light in this office. It's way too dark here."

Jason rose from his chair, walked around his desk, reached out his hand, and with a brilliant smile said, "Maybe you're right Chuck. And maybe you're not. But it sure is good to see you."

Chuck took Jason's hand with mouth open. He had come to expect a tight-lipped, somewhat stiff and cold financial advisor who never cracked a smile. And here was Jason welcoming him like a long lost friend. "Amazing!" he thought.

At that instant, the same word entered Jason's mind, though for different reasons. "Amazing," he thought. "I used to create this man as an arrogant fool. Now I'm just creating him as a guy named Chuck who has a few irritating quirks but who maybe now I can get to know a bit better."

I hope you will take a lesson from Jason. If there is somebody out there who, for some reason, you've labeled negatively, realize that it is you who applied the label. Consider what possibilities might arise if you were to remove that label and just accept the person for who he or she is.

EXERCISES FOR PRINCIPLE 3: ACCEPTANCE

Exercise 1: *Understand How Non-Acceptance and Acceptance Affect You*

We have all had to deal with situations that were hard to accept. The objective of this exercise is for you to recall several of those situations in order to better understand how non-acceptance affected you emotionally, and how acceptance did or could have affected you. The overall purpose is for you to understand better how the Principle of Acceptance can affect your reaction to events in your life.

First, consider this list of twenty emotion concepts:

angry	frustrated	sad	disappointed
fearful	anxious	guilty	ashamed
confused	betrayed	resentful	powerless
cheated	deceived	lonely	disgusted
exhausted	intimidated	discouraged	victimized

Next, recall three times in your life when you have encountered situations that were stressful. These could have been events at work, home, school, or somewhere else. They could have concerned family, finances, thwarted plans, health, your job, problems with friends, or some other area. For each of the three situations, choose three words listed above that best describe how you felt when you first encountered the situation:

Situation 1: _____ _____ _____

Situation 2: _____ _____ _____

Situation 3: _____ _____ _____

Now, for each situation, recall at what point you came to fully emotionally accept its reality. Or, if you never came to accept the situation fully, imagine that you did accept it. Reflect on how your emotions changed when you applied the Principle of Acceptance, or how they would have changed if you had applied it. For each event, did one of the three emotions you listed disappear most fully and quickly when you emotionally accepted the situation? If so, which one?

Situation 1: _____

Situation 2: _____

Situation 3: _____

Exercise 2: *Apply the Principle of Acceptance to Others*

We all know what it's like to negatively categorize someone in our lives. In fact, most of us have probably done that very thing recently with someone we know. If you are an exception, then congratulations for living by the Principle of Acceptance as you deal with others in your life. For the rest of us—including me once in a while, I must admit—it might be valuable to reflect on how we could be more accepting of all others who travel with us down the River of Life. This exercise is meant to aid in that reflection.

Think of someone you know who you have mentally labeled with one or more negative concepts. List one, two, or three of these labels in the spaces provided:

_____   _____   _____

Next, list the kinds of behavior that led you to apply that label or labels to the person:

_____

_____

Now, do you think that the label or labels that color your thoughts about the person are the only way in which to interpret those behaviors? Write down some other ways those behaviors might be interpreted:

_____

_____

_____

Finally, take several minutes to reflect carefully on this person. What are some of the person's positive qualities? What behaviors, attitudes, ideas, accomplishments, activities, relationships, or other characteristics of the person go beyond the negative label or labels you applied to him or her and attest to the person's fuller reality? Write these down:

_____

_____

_____

_____

_____

_____

_____

_____

_____

Does completing this exercise lead you to think of the other person in a more comprehensive and positive way?

Can you think of anyone else you know who you have also labeled negatively? If so, go through this exercise again with that person in mind.

PRINCIPLE 4

☙

Thought

Make Thinking Your Powerful Ally

*"Great men are they who see that spiritual is stronger than
any material force, that thoughts rule the world."*
Ralph Waldo Emerson
from *Letters and Social Aims*

Our thoughts can be our most powerful ally, or our worst enemy. They can lift us on wings of freedom or act as a ball and chain, causing us to shuffle through our days.

Our thoughts include our beliefs, attitudes, imaginings, and perceptions. These are all part of an ongoing stream of consciousness that carries us along on its current each day from the moment we wake until we fall asleep. Most of us are usually so deeply immersed in our stream of consciousness that we rarely reflect on it. But when we do, it becomes evident that it affects every aspect of our lives.

In the case of physical health, the power of thought is clear. Negative, defeatist beliefs and attitudes can ravage our body by fueling stress, weakening our immune system, and promoting substance abuse. On the other hand, our thoughts can work with our physiology to foster healing. As a physician, I have seen this repeatedly. Some patients see a diagnosis of cancer or heart trouble as a death sentence. They slump into a resigned outlook that erodes their will to overcome the malady. Others view the diagnosis as a reason to learn about the ailment, renew bonds with friends and family, and move forward determined to beat the disease. Outcomes for these two groups are often very different due to the healing power of positive thoughts.

Core Beliefs

Our core beliefs—our most basic convictions about the world and ourselves—have an especially powerful effect on all aspects of our wellness. These core beliefs are so deeply embedded in our psyche that they dictate our overall attitude toward life. In doing so, they also govern the character of the world we experience. For example, some people are convinced that the world is an unfriendly, inhospitable place. Accordingly, they assume a pessimistic, cynical attitude toward whatever they encounter. This, in turn, has a stultifying effect on their behaviors, relationships, and other aspects of their lives. The end result is that they find themselves actually living in a rather inhospitable world.

Others have a very different conviction about the nature of reality. They view the world as a garden of opportunity, a playground for creating happy relationships and striving for heartfelt goals. These people tend to approach reality with optimistic, confident attitudes and behaviors. As a result, they find themselves living in a world that for the most part conforms to their core belief.

Some might scoff at the idea that we create the character of the world we encounter. They might claim that aside from anyone's thought processes, reality actually is a rather mean and hostile place, as shown by its potential dangers and malicious people. In reply, I admit that we should be careful crossing streets. And certainly, there are unscrupulous individuals who would take advantage of us if they could. However, this does not mean that reality itself is hateful, but only that we must approach it judiciously. The world also contains countless wonders and bounteous pleasures. And the vast majority of our neighbors are decent and kind people who will respond to a positive outlook with positive reactions.

But if the character of the reality we experience is determined by our thought processes, does this mean that the world in itself is actually neutral—a kind of blank canvas on which we apply our mental paint? No. My conviction is that in itself, apart from our thoughts, reality is not neutral at all, but is permeated with loving Spirit. Those who perceive the world as hospitable are much closer to the truth than those who do not. Evidence that reality is ultimately benevolent is provided by the fact that it tends to reward people who embrace it with their positive thoughts and attitudes. Doing so creates a kind of self-fulfilling prophecy by opening paths for love, accomplishment, and fulfillment.

The Law of Attraction

The idea of a self-fulfilling prophecy is taken a step further by the Law of Attraction, which states that people receive what they focus on with their minds. If we constantly worry about failure, failure is more likely to happen. If we continually focus on being a success, success will be almost assured.

Within limits, there is truth in the Law of Attraction. For example, if you go to a job interview thinking of all the ways you could fail the interview, your nerves will probably work against you, dulling your shine. But if you go in convinced that you will impress the interviewer favorably, you are more likely to do that very thing and get the job. Or suppose your dream is to become a doctor. If you believe you wouldn't be able to succeed in medical school, you probably won't even take the first steps toward fulfilling your dream. But if you make up your mind that the world will give you what you want if you work hard for it, then there is a good chance you will become the doctor you want to be.

The Law of Attraction has been around for a century or more. Some people explain why it works by saying that when we believe it, reality changes to accommodate us. That may sometimes be true. But belief in the Law of Attraction can also lead *us* to change to accommodate reality. It does this by promoting attitudes and actions that move us toward our goals. In any event, belief in the Law of Attraction can work wonders. That's not to say you can simply sprawl in your easy chair, thinking over and over, "I'm going to become a doctor!" or "I'm going to become a great writer!" You have to work hard at whatever you want to accomplish. But generating a strong belief that life will give you what you ask is a powerful strategy for success.

In light of all this, a question arises: if reality rewards those who approach it with a welcoming attitude, does it punish those who approach it with negativity? No, reality does not punish us, no more than the orchard punishes those who refuse to enjoy its fruits. It is we who punish ourselves if we alienate ourselves from the world through our core beliefs. We do our lives much harm if we think that reality is somehow our opponent. It is not. The power of belief is so strong that thinking of life in that way sours our attitudes, limits our choices, and estranges us from people. Those who think life is against them will, by those very thoughts, shut themselves out of many of the world's gifts. In this way, they will tend to find what they expect.

Who Am I?

Our most fundamental core beliefs concern who we essentially are—our self-image. Like other core beliefs, our self-image was largely determined when we were children. Our parents and others led us to think of ourselves in certain ways: as being capable, lovable, and infinitely valuable, or as being more or less deficient. Those lessons often linger throughout our lives, either brightening or dulling our experiences.

Our self-image and our core beliefs about the world tend to wax and wane together, as reality reflects back to us how we view ourselves. If we regard ourselves as weak, unworthy, or unable to fulfill our dreams, the world will respond accordingly, seeming to confirm our belief. But if we see ourselves as strong, worthy, and capable, here too the world will react in accordance with our convictions. This is another case where our core beliefs serve as self-fulfilling prophecies, especially for beliefs about our capabilities. As Henry Ford remarked, "Whether you think you can or you think you can't, you're usually right."

How Defining Themselves Affects the Lives of Tamara and Cindy

Our thoughts about who we are may vary between negative and positive, but many people show an affinity for one pole or the other. This is illustrated by two thirty-something women, Tamara and Cindy.

Tamara often lingers on limiting beliefs such as that she is plain, a klutz, and doomed to be a failure at anything beyond the most ordinary. If you tried to convince her otherwise, you would have a hard go of it. The result is that she is timid, unusually self-conscious, and very resistant to change. She never takes risks and is always careful to say only what she thinks people want to hear. Her belief that she is essentially weak also affects her health, as she easily succumbs to whatever "bug" is making the rounds. And her self-consciousness has a stultifying effect on her social life because she has difficulty feeling comfortable enough to genuinely go out to other people. In sum, Tamara identifies so closely with her negative beliefs that she acts out in her life what she is convinced she is, an unremarkable, relatively weak person. And this acting out, in turn, adversely affects many aspects of her wellness.

Cindy, in contrast, tends to have thoughts and images of herself as being strong and competent. If someone tried to convince Cindy that she is mistaken in her self-regard, the words would, thankfully, go in one ear and out the other. She understands that to fulfill her dreams, she sometimes has to leave her comfort zone, and she is willing to do that when necessary. She is friendly and likable, but she isn't afraid to speak her mind when she feels it is right, which is a trait that leads other people to respect her. Her vision of herself as strong also has a health benefit, as she tends to recuperate quickly in the rare instances when she catches a cold or the flu. Overall, Cindy identifies so completely with her core beliefs in herself that she has no doubt that she is what she believes herself to be, a strong and competent woman.

On one level, Tamara and Cindy are both right: each is what she defines herself to be. And each woman's degree of success and happiness in life will be affected strongly by those beliefs. Through her actions, Tamara will attempt to prove to herself and the world the truth of her beliefs about her limited abilities. Unfortunately, she will probably succeed. Cindy, on the other hand, will show through her actions that she is indeed strong and competent.

On a more basic level, however, Cindy's core belief about herself is much closer than Tamara's to capturing the reality of who she is—her True Self.

The True Self is an ancient and revered spiritual concept that begins with the idea that no definition can capture a person's essence because every person has infinite potentiality. We humans are the only kind of being that can define—and redefine—ourselves any way we want. A person can be a mail deliverer for thirty years and then decide to become a singer (or designer or psychiatric nurse). Or she can be a singer for thirty years and then decide to become a mail deliverer. It is up to each of us what we are to be and become. There is no limit. But through all of the definitions we may give ourselves, as son, sister, parent, student, employee, manager, singer, mail deliverer, and on and on, one central part of us remains unchanged. This is our True Self. For example, I define myself, among other things, as a husband, parent, physician, and a man with a touch of arthritis in his shoulder. But I also know that I would still exist even if none of these had been true. This part of myself that exists apart from all definitions of me is my core, my essence, my True Self.

Tamara's problem is that she identifies strongly with her definition of herself as being weak, plain, and limited. She can't see past this definition. She can't see that it is only her thoughts that are creating herself as limited. If she could grasp the idea of the True Self, she would realize that in actuality, she has no limits. She can define herself anyway she wants. Her self-definition would change—and *she* would change.

Assume Responsibility, Not Blame

Despite the tendency of negative core beliefs to create major stumbling blocks in our lives, we must not blame anyone, including ourselves, for having such beliefs. Core beliefs usually stem from childhood, when brains are very malleable. Families, teachers, peers, and society mold children's thoughts to reflect their own ideas about the basic nature of reality. Parents are especially influential, and sometimes teach their children negative outlooks. Other kids become cynical about the world through experiencing childhood abuse or deprivation. Such beliefs may become so deeply embedded that as adults we are unconscious of them even though they guide our attitudes and actions. And we cannot be blamed for any beliefs, conscious or not, helpful or harmful, that came from being indoctrinated as children.

But blame is not the same thing as responsibility. Blaming someone for something is a moral judgment, but to assign responsibility for something is simply to identify its cause. Even if some of our core beliefs were programmed into us when we were children, as adults we are ultimately the source of our own beliefs. This means that in the end, how each person experiences reality falls squarely on his or her shoulders. If the world appears to you to be basically inhospitable, unkind, unfair, or hostile, you are the one who, through your thoughts and attitudes, are creating that character in the world you experience. And you are free to change it. You need not settle for any pattern of thinking or behavior that you have fallen into, no matter how it initially arose. For each of us, our core beliefs need not be dead weight that we drag through our lives as we feel sorry for ourselves and blame the world for our situation. As adults, we are capable of erupting out of our old ways of thinking and reframing reality.

Spiritual Perspectives: A World Suffused with Loving Spirit

A powerful way to defuse harmful core beliefs is to replace them with broad spiritual perspectives. The main premise of this book is that spiritual ideas promote wellness in all dimensions of our being. They do this by providing a comprehensive framework that helps us make sense of our lives. When we first encounter a spiritual truth or principle, it takes form in our mind as a thought. If we accept the principle, it becomes a belief that can influence other thoughts, as well as our attitudes and behavior. In time, the principle may become a core belief. At that point it will have a profound positive effect on our attitudes, actions, and well-being.

You have already encountered several spiritual principles. In the first chapter, you learned about a fundamental Ayurvedic belief:

Wellness requires balancing our inner nature with outer nature.

In the second chapter you were introduced to the fundamental Principle of Calmness. In the third chapter, I explained another spiritual belief, which, in one form or another, has been a basic part of every great religious tradition, the Principle of Acceptance:

Don't fight emotionally against the River of Life, but let its flow empower you.

In the present chapter we are learning that the Principle of Thought implies several important spiritual ideas that go hand-in-hand with the earlier ones:

When we open our arms to the world, the world responds with its own embrace.
Your True Self has no limits.
We cannot be blamed for what we were led to believe as children.
But as adults, we must take responsibility for our core beliefs.

Finally, there is this basic spiritual belief, the source and foundation for all the others:

Reality is suffused with loving Spirit.

The belief that we live in a world brimming with Spirit underlies this book. If you ponder this profound idea, it will help you understand more deeply the other principles you learn about here. And you will see that they are all interconnected and mutually supporting.

More important, if you then go further and allow this most fundamental principle to become a core belief, it will make an enormous positive difference in your experience. When you envision the world as being full of opportunity, beauty, love, and wonder, these thoughts will reverberate in your life. Spirit itself will settle into your thoughts, and its gentle but enormous power will infuse all aspects of your being. At that point the world will become—

Spirit Manifests Itself in How We Think of Others

In one of my blog entries at www.DrRaj.com I told of going to a presentation by a friend, a young woman who had spent considerable time in India teaching self-empowerment to sex workers, mostly females, in the red-light areas of Kolkata. I was inspired to write the blog because of what one of the sex workers had told my friend: "I am the same as you, but I will do anything to feed my children, whose father they do not know."

As I reflected on the words, "I am the same as you," I was struck by the thought that though seemingly false on the surface, they were profoundly true on a deep spiritual level. They were true because Shakti, the Divine Feminine principle, the source of creativity, resides in all women, regardless of socio-economic condition, caste, race, occupation, or age. An aging sex worker sitting on a curb, hoping some man will choose her so she can make some money to feed her children, has no less a claim to Divine Femininity than any other woman.

To think of women in this way, to recognize the presence of Spirit in each one, entails treating all women with respect, for that is truly honoring Spirit. Here we see again how our thoughts can make a profound difference in our attitudes, our actions, our lives.

more fully than ever before—your home, your playground, your field of dreams, where you can find success and fulfillment in many aspects of living.

But for this most basic principle and all the others to do their wonderful work, it is not enough simply to think about them for a moment or two and then move on. You must read, reread, and ponder them. You must attempt to understand how the different principles are related and mutually support each other. You must make them a central part of your thinking.

Do that in any way that works for you. Write them down. Put them on cards you review every morning when you rise, and every night before bed. Mark up this book (if you own it!) with your own comments about them. Talk to your friends and family about them. Meditate on them. Perhaps most helpful, observe what happens in your daily life and understand how their truth is exhibited there again and again.

Whatever methods you use, just *seize* them with your mind.

EXERCISES FOR PRINCIPLE 4: THOUGHT

Exercise 1: *Overcome Negative Self-Ascriptions*

There are many causes for negative self-beliefs and many ways they can arise. Negative self-ascriptions typically go hand-in-hand with irrational thoughts that seem to confirm them. For example, your thinking may exaggerate the importance of criticisms or events that you judge as negative, while at the same time your thoughts may minimize the significance of positive events or compliments. You may be jumping to unjustified conclusions that put you in a negative light, or you may think that it is necessary to be perfect in some of area of life in order to feel good about yourself. Another kind of irrational thought is to continually define yourself in relation to some quality in others such as their popularity or accomplishments. Whatever form they take, a proven method for dealing with such thoughts is to identify and challenge them.

Your exercise is to practice doing this. For three entire days, commit yourself to observing and recording in a notebook small enough for your pocket or purse any negative self-ascriptions you find in your thinking as you go about your daily activities. Whenever you find yourself entertaining a self-defeating thought such as "I can't do this," "I should be more like so-and-so," or "I'm not attractive," write it down. Then challenge the thought by asking yourself what is the evidence you actually have for the thought and whether you are jumping to conclusions, making unwarranted assumptions, or exaggerating. Then write down a substitute thought that serves to contradict or otherwise defuse the negative one, and insert the new thought into your mental repertoire. For example, if the negative thought is, "I should be more like so-and-so," then, as a substitute, think or say to yourself, "I am a worthwhile and whole person as I am, and I should be myself and only myself at all times."

Do this for three days and then look for patterns in any negative self-ascriptions that you identify. Doing this will strengthen your ability to identify negative thoughts about yourself at the moment they occur. You are also likely to develop a set of positive self-ascriptions that you can substitute for the negative ones when they occur.

Exercise 2: *Experience Your True Self*

It is difficult to define your True Self except negatively. Your True Self is what is left over when all other self-definitions have been stripped away. The intent of this exercise is to guide you in taking some steps toward realizing the reality of your True Self.

Your first step is to make a list of all the ways you define yourself. Your list might include, for example, the following words: woman, daughter, wife, mother, aunt, cousin, design consultant, member of the PTA, Christian, middle-aged person, vegetarian, chief cook and bottle washer, skier, Californian, yoga practitioner, art aficionado, and so on. Make the list as long as you can, full of the many ways you can describe yourself.

Your second step in the exercise is to devise an alternative for each of the self-defining words you have listed. For example, for "woman" put down "man," and imagine you were born a man, but that this person is still you. Likewise, put down alternatives such as: son, husband, father, uncle, second cousin, architect, member of the Elks, Jewish, young person, meat-eater, yard and auto up-keeper, tennis player, New Yorker, Tai chi practitioner, history buff, and so on. For a few minutes, imagine that you yourself are a person who fits that new set of descriptive words.

For your third step, imagine that none of the definitions from either list is true of you, but that you still somehow exist. Imagine that you are neither a woman nor a man and that you fulfill no descriptive word on either list. This includes imagining that you also do not have a body. Then ask yourself, what would be left of you if this were true? What core essence would be left? That core essence is who you are apart from any and all definitions. It is your True Self. You are unable to define this core essence directly because you have thrown away all lists, all words that could be used to do so. Yet it is there.

Some consider their True Self to be their soul. Others identify the True Self as being the experiencer—that part of you that is the source and subject of all of your experiences. Obviously, this experiencer cannot itself be an object of any experience. Yet somehow we catch a glimmer of its existence and know that it is there, that it must be there.

After you strip away all definitions and descriptions of you and squarely face the question of what remains, you may be able to catch a glimmer of your True Self. If and when you do, contemplate the truth of the statement, "You have infinite potential to define yourself, because at your core you are undefined, open, and full of possibility."

PRINCIPLE 5

 C3

Dharma

Find Your Passion and Purpose

"Hold fast to dreams
For if dreams die
Life is a broken-winged bird
That cannot fly."

Langston Hughes
from the poem "Dreams"

Many spiritual traditions hold that we are each designed for some special purpose. For example, Christianity teaches that God has a specific plan for each of us. The idea is also present in the Hindu belief that every person has a proper path in life—their *dharma*—that depends on their inner nature. To find and follow your dharma is to let your inner nature shine forth and determine your hopes, dreams, and long-term purpose. Your purpose may be to become an excellent manager, mechanic, physician, chef, or parent. Or it might be to fulfill any of ten thousand other roles. But whatever it may be, it is essential to understand your dharma and then follow it.

Why is it essential? Because there is only one you, and there will never be another. You bring a unique combination of talents, experience, interests, and personality to the world, a blend that has never existed before and will never exist again. And because you are special, because you are one of a kind, you have a purpose in this life that only you can fulfill.

Accepting that We Have a Special Purpose

Some who read this will immediately respond that there is nothing special about them. But I refuse to believe that. Tragically, countless people are led to accept such a false story when they are children by insensitive adults or peers. They then carry that absurd "lesson" into adulthood.

Others, more fortunate, may grow up with considerable self-regard, but the end result is the same. Caught up in the responsibilities of adulthood, they find themselves working for a paycheck at a job that fits their nature poorly. In time, they come to define themselves by that work. Their youthful dreams fade away, and they begin feeling "ordinary." But the truth is, not one of us is ordinary. We are each special, with a unique combination of aptitudes, temperament, and passions that help make us the individuals we are. This includes you. And out of your singular nature, you have something that *only you* can offer the world.

So please reject any suggestion that you are not special. Embrace wholeheartedly the fact that you are one of a kind. The Principle of Dharma asks you to understand your unique qualities, seek out what is highest and deepest in you, and grasp your true nature. When you do so, you will discover your purpose in life if you have not done so already. If you do not seek what is special in you and learn how you can contribute uniquely to humanity and our beautiful planet, you will do yourself and the entire world a disfavor.

I sometimes compare finding and following your dharma to locating and buying a pair of shoes that are perfect for you in size, material, color, and style. The shoes prove themselves to be comfortable, serviceable, and aesthetically right for you, and you love to put them on and wear them each day. In contrast, not following your dharma is like wearing a pair of shoes that are too tight or too loose, shoes that pinch your toes or rub your heels raw, or whose color or style grates on your eyes. When wearing such shoes, we tend to feel out of sync. Likewise, when we do not follow our dharma, our lives feel out of kilter. Consciously or unconsciously, we know we have a true calling that we are not paying attention to, and this knowledge creates uneasiness throughout our being.

This deep discomfort comes from several sources. Part of it is because we realize, even if only subconsciously, that by not allowing our talents and interests to determine our path in life, we are being false to ourselves. Being true to self requires understanding who we are. And this includes understanding our true interests and talents and then acting on that knowledge.

The unease also comes from the fact that an essential component of happiness is to apply ourselves to long-term goals that personally matter to us. By aiming for objectives that fulfill our natural passions, we infuse our lives with great meaning. We also foster personal growth by challenging ourselves to make the most of our aptitudes and interests. This creates an active, purposeful life based on our deepest motivations. If we never dare to challenge ourselves, then our talents lie fallow and we stagnate. But if we let our inner nature direct us to a life of meaningful achievement, we grow, we develop, we become.

Finally, our discomfort comes from a lack of balance in our lives that affects our overall wellness. The four-dimensional view says that total wellness is a matter of harmonizing all of our dimensions. When we do not pursue long-range goals that arise from our inner nature, we shortchange both our mental and spiritual aspects. The result is a disharmony that may also have repercussions in our physical and social dimensions.

Understanding Your Purpose

Many people never discover and fill their proper role in life. One main reason is that they find themselves traveling down a road on which they feel trapped. They may realize the work they are doing doesn't suit their natural aptitudes and passions, but they can't see a way out. They may spend years, even a lifetime, at jobs that seem pointless to them except for providing a paycheck. In actuality, there are many other roads branching out from the one they are on, directions that would better fit their personality and talents, roads they could be passionate about. Yet they may be barely aware of those alternatives. They feel imprisoned, but their "prison" is created by their lack of self-knowledge, imagination, and will. They don't realize that no matter what path they are on, or where they are in their lives, other pathways always exist. And they can always make a choice to look deep into themselves, discover what purpose they are best suited for, and then set out in a direction that will realize their natural potential.

To understand whether you are following your dharma, ask yourself a simple question: Would you continue doing your present work if you suddenly became wealthy? If your answer is "Yes," you are probably following your dharma right now. If it is "No," you are not. Ask a designer who loves to design clothes if she would stop designing just because she became wealthy, and she will reply, "Why should I stop doing the thing that fills my days with pleasure and my life with meaning, just because of an influx of money?" Ask many others, such as artists, scientists, gardeners, teachers, or craftspeople the same question and you will get a similar answer. If they were to win millions in the lottery, they would likely use some of the money to make their work even more satisfying. I see the teacher who loves teaching using a portion of the money to create her own school. I see the gardener who is passionate about growing things buying land and then designing and helping to create a neighborhood park.

Somewhere inside, you know whether or not you are following your dharma. Do you feel you are being all you could be? Are you seizing life by setting long-range goals that are deeply meaningful to you? If the answer is "No," it is time to start trying to understand what your dharma is. This may be difficult because it requires contemplation, and in today's society self-knowledge can be hard to gain. There are more and more diversions that keep people on the surface of things: television and movies, newspapers and magazines, online social networks, shopping, and more. All of these may be enjoyable, but they may also keep us from digging deep into ourselves and realizing where our destiny lies.

Fortunately, there are some tools you can use to get in touch with what would create passion and purpose in your life. For one thing, it can help to re-imagine the dreams you had in childhood of what you wanted to become as an adult. As a child, you may have sensed the road that would best suit you. But as you matured and the cares of the world fell on your shoulders, you may have lost that understanding. By returning in your imagination to what gave you joy in childhood, you may uncover important clues about what would give you joy in the future.

Another tool is to ask yourself, "What is my passion?" Or what would it be if you were free to pursue any objective at all? Perhaps you greatly enjoy a particular kind of endeavor. If so, that is reason enough to explore that road further in thought and imagination. The kind of purpose you should be looking for is work that feeds your innermost being. Ask yourself again what you would do if you suddenly won millions in a lottery. But this time, think hard about how you would spend the rest of your life if you were wealthy. If you didn't have to worry about a paycheck but could do some kind of work just for the love of it, what would that work be? Engaging in such thought experiments can help uncover what your deepest interests are.

As you investigate your dharma, remember to seek a life purpose that does not harm others but rather lifts them up. Unfortunately, many

The Self-Doubter and the Self-Affirmer

Even after discovering what purpose you are perfectly suited for, you may find your proposed new pathway strewn with obstacles created by the Self-Doubter. The Self-Doubter is nothing more than negative self-beliefs that act like speed bumps to slow your progress or even stop your journey altogether. It's the opposite of the Self-Affirmer, which acts like a road grader to clear those speed bumps away.

I heard the admonitions of the Self-Doubter when I began my journey into becoming a healer not just of Body but of all four dimensions. Its insistent voice whispered to me that I should stay with what I knew about. What did I know about holistic medicine? What did I know about spirituality? Who was I to think I could make a difference in this area?

The insidious voice of the Self-Doubter sometimes made me wonder whether I was on the right path, but I steeled myself against its negativity, and at the same time fed and strengthened my Self-Affirmer. As I made progress down my chosen pathway the Self-Doubter's voice got weaker and weaker while the Self-Affirmer's got increasingly strong. This struggle helped me understand very well how fulfilling one's purpose is intimately related to the power of belief that we learned about in the last chapter.

Don't let your Self-Doubter throw obstacles onto your path. Let your Self-Affirmer push the mental obstacles aside and create a level road toward achieving your goals.

people pursue goals that worsen the lives of others because their main objective is to gratify their ego by seeking money, power, or possessions are rewards that often accompany fulfillment, but they are secondary. To walk a road of purpose that is also spiritual is to walk a road with Heart. And as you know, the dimension of Heart is about caring for and respecting our fellow inhabitants on earth. To find and follow your dharma is to take a journey that engages your entire being in *all four* dimensions. When your goals reverberate strongly within your Mind, Body, Spirit and Heart, you know you are on the right path for you.

Setting out on a New Path

It is one thing to understand your dharma. It is another to follow it. Even if there are signs that a road was built just for you, it can take courage to start down it. Fear can keep us from acting: fear of the unknown, fear of losing what we have, fear of failure. Though we may realize that we are not being true to ourselves, we remain stuck in old, half-hearted ways.

But fear is almost always overblown. Fear is like stress. It has its purpose in motivating action when there is something in the neighborhood that is a true threat. But most of the things we fear are not actually dangerous in themselves. And sometimes we fear what is good for us—like children afraid of an inoculation that will lead to better health. What overcomes fear is action. The best antidote for a woman perched for the first time on the end of a diving board, shaking with trepidation, is not to keep standing there imagining disaster but to jump or dive in and discover with her own body that the water is forgiving.

This is not to say that in starting out on a new path we must burn our bridges behind us. That may work for some people, but for many an all-or-nothing approach would be wrong. It may lead them to feel they must achieve immediate success on the new path, and this can result in a great deal of stress.

Eric's Judicious Path to Fulfilling His Dream

For most people, a more judicious approach may be appropriate. This is illustrated very well by the story of a young man I will call Eric.

Eric worked in a convenience store from noon to eight p.m. five days a week. He greatly enjoyed cooking for his friends, and they always raved about what a great chef he was. Realizing that cooking was what he loved most to do, Eric started dreaming of owning a restaurant. But that seemed impossible on his income, so he wondered how else he might express his love for cooking.

One day at the convenience store, he started thinking about the many people who came in at lunchtime to buy a wrapped sandwich and a bag of chips. He knew the sandwiches weren't fresh and not of high quality. He was sure he could do better. So why not go into the sandwich making business?

The more he entertained this idea, the more attractive it seemed. Building up his courage, he started visiting small local bakeries to ask if he could, for a price, use one of their tables and an oven in the morning to bake bread. After several tries, he found one that agreed. He started going to the bakery at six a.m. with fresh meat, vegetables, flour, and other ingredients he had bought the evening before and kept in his refrigerator. He would then bake fresh, hot bread and make twenty ham, turkey, and roast beef sandwiches. After wrapping the sandwiches, he placed them in lined bags and at nine a.m. started visiting nearby offices, giving workers free samples. He also gave them a business card with his cell number if they wanted to order sandwiches delivered to their office the next day. Right away, people started calling to tell him how wonderful his sandwiches were and to place orders. Within one week he was delivering thirty sandwiches a day starting at eleven a.m., and then hurrying to his job at the convenience store. He also continued giving out free sandwiches in the morning. Within two weeks, he had hired another person to help deliver the sandwiches. Within two months, he had two delivery people. All that time, he kept putting in his hours at the convenience store. Finally, three months after he started, he realized that even after expenses, he was making more money from his sandwich business than from his other job, and he handed in his resignation.

Eric's story demonstrates that a daring and proactive approach to launching oneself into a new path can also be judicious. He didn't give up his job until he had found considerable success following his dharma. That required long hours each day. For three months, he worked nearly eighty hours a week. But half that time he was following his dream by doing something he loved, so was it work or not?

This brings up another main reason that some people, even if they dream of setting out on a new path that would fit their interests and talents better, never do so: inertia. We all have our comfort zones, and it can be hard to leave them. Setting out in a new direction—even if it stirs our passion—can be difficult, demanding work. And many people are reluctant to give up their comfort. What they may not realize is that setting out on their true path would energize and enrich their lives immeasurably.

Eric's story also illustrates another important point—the fact that it can be OK to temper your aspirations to fit realities. Eric's initial dream was to own a restaurant, but he felt that would be impossible given his present circumstances. So he chose a different path that would still express his inner nature and would have a better chance of success in the near term. Another person might have chosen to continue working and save his money over several years to buy part ownership in a small café. Either choice could be a viable dharma, as long as it expressed the individual's inner nature and passion.

In fact, any movement to fulfill your dharma, however small, is much better than none. This is illustrated by Janine, a forty-year-old woman who as a teen had dreamed of being a veterinarian.

Janine's Path to Fulfilling Her Dream

Janine had completed two years of college, aiming for a veterinary degree. But due to circumstances, she had dropped out and started working as a bank teller. After twenty years, she was now a loan officer. Though she found some satisfaction in her job, she still looked longingly at any veterinary office she passed by, wondering what would have happened if she had continued following her dream.

Though she was a lover of animals, Janine didn't have any since she lived in an apartment building that didn't allow pets. One day she noticed a sign on a bulletin board asking for volunteers to work at the local Society for the Prevention of Cruelty to Animals. She doubted she had any extra time to offer, but the cause seemed such a good one that she took down the phone number and next day called. Soon she was volunteering her time on Saturday afternoons.

Janine found quickly that caring for dogs, cats, and other animals that had found their way to the shelter was immensely satisfying. She also came into contact with several veterinarians and decided to start applying for a job at a veterinary hospital. Though she had to take a substantial cut in pay, three months later she was working as a veterinary assistant. Soon, she was also enrolled at night in a four-year program that would eventually lead to an associate veterinarian position.

Good for Janine! Even if taking the volunteer position was all she ever did to fulfill her dharma, she would have done herself an immense favor. As it turned out, her exposure to something she loved also gave her the knowledge, imagination, and will to move much farther down that path with confidence and determination.

There is much more that could be said about finding and following your dharma path, but the main message of this principle is simple: learn what will give your life its greatest meaning and purpose, and then go for it. As you walk your dharma path, plan well and wisely. And do not forget to make thought your powerful ally, as belief is the fuel that powers the engine of action. If you believe strongly in your dreams and in yourself, you are already beginning to create those dreams in reality. The bottom line is that your life is a great adventure. You have the power to determine the nature of that adventure by choosing a road with heart, passion, and purpose that fits your unique talents and interests. When you make that choice, your journey will become exciting, joyful, and profound.

EXERCISES FOR PRINCIPLE 5: DHARMA

Exercise 1: *Discover Your Unique Purpose*

Those who have already found the path to accomplishment that best suits them are sure to feel excited by their work and by performing it with excellence. Others have yet to find the path that suits them best. If you are among the latter group, this exercise is designed to help you discover your unique purpose.

You will need to set aside a little time on four consecutive days, probably no more than a half to one hour. The first day is for brainstorming. Find a place where you can think undisturbed. Using a notebook or computer, make a list of every job, career, or pursuit you've ever worked at or ever thought or fantasized that you might enjoy. Include dreams you had as a child and teenager, even if they seem silly to you now. Include not just jobs and careers, but pursuits you have enjoyed or thought you would enjoy—stamp collecting, hiking, skiing, solving puzzles, traveling, anything at all that attracts you. If you let your mind roam freely and brainstorm without censoring your thoughts, you will likely end with a long list. After completing the list, set it aside until the next day.

The second day is for reviewing and shortening your list. Look at each item carefully and decide how attractive it seems to you relative to the other items. That should be your only criterion, not how "ridiculous" or "impossible" it may seem. Select 12 items on your list that are the most attractive to you. Once you have done that, go through the list again, carefully and thoughtfully. Cut the list further in half, until you find the six items that are most attractive to you.

The third day is for doing one more cut. Reflect on each of the items that remain on your list and reduce them down to the three jobs, careers, or kinds of work that are most attractive to you. Now, close your eyes and visualize yourself doing each kind of work. Try to feel what it would be like to do the work. Then send a message to your subconscious mind to consider each of the three items left on your list and to choose which one suits you best. Instruct it to give you an answer by the next day. It is perfectly all right if, during the next twenty-four hours, you also consciously entertain the three items in an attempt to determine which one best suits and most excites you. That way, both your conscious and unconscious mind are working on the problem. Fully expect that within twenty-four hours, you will become certain, either gradually or in a sudden epiphany, which of your top three jobs, careers, or pursuits is best designed for you.

If you don't get the answer in twenty-four hours, then keep at it. Keep telling your subconscious mind to give you the answer you need, and keep expecting that answer to come to you. Just keep at it until you find yourself with the answer.

Once you have settled on your true calling, your dharma road, go on to the next exercise.

Exercise 2: *Create a Plan for Achieving Your Purpose; then Work the Plan*

Assuming that you either have found your unique purpose by completing the first exercise or you already suspect what your purpose is but have so far been unable to move far down that pathway, this exercise is intended to assist you in moving toward fulfilling your purpose.

Develop a Mission Statement. Your first step is to write down, as fully but succinctly as you can, a mission statement that describes what fulfilling your purpose would amount to. For example, one person might write the following: "My mission is to become a best-selling fiction author." Another might write, "My mission is to develop a successful plumbing business." A third person might write, "My mission is to become the best elementary school teacher I can become."

Develop an Overall Plan for Fulfilling Your Mission Statement. Here, address the issue of how to go about fulfilling your purpose, your dream. What steps must you take to get you there? Write them down clearly, and number them. The rationale here is to get you thinking about the practical issues involved in moving down your path. Devote one part of your plan to listing obstacles you may have to overcome at each step and how you can overcome them. Devote another part of your plan to listing the resources you have or can call on to help you fulfill your plan.

Develop a Detailed Daily To-do List for Each Step of Your Plan. Here's where you get down into the details of your plan by determining what you can do today and each day thereafter to put into action your plan to fulfill your purpose. Realize that each day you can do something, even if it takes only a few minutes, to help complete one of the steps in your plan. To that end, and to keep you on target, set aside sufficient time each Sunday evening to write down a detailed To-Do list of what you will accomplish each day of the coming week to make your plan come alive. Then consult the list each day and carry out the To-Do's for that day.

Don't give excuses to yourself for not working your plan. Don't complain that you're working at a job that takes all your time. And don't use the excuse that the obstacles that stand in the way of your fulfilling your purpose are just too great. You were built to overcome obstacles. Remember the saying of Lao-tzu, "The journey of a thousand miles begins with a single step." That's as true for you as for anyone else. One of the keys to getting where you want to go is to **start**. Another key is to **keep on moving**. Every day, there is almost always some small task that will take only an hour or less, maybe only five or ten minutes, that will get you a step further down the pathway to fulfilling your mission statement and your purpose.

Now, how does it feel finally to be on your way?

❧

The Virtues of Heart

Practice Love, Compassion, and Kindness

*"This is my simple religion. There is no need
for temples; no need for complicated
philosophy. Our own brain, our own heart
is our temple; the philosophy is kindness."*

The Dalai Lama
quoted in *The Dalai Lama: A Policy of Kindness,* by S. Piburn

Spirit enters our lives in countless ways. It touches our body through the cool, refreshing taste of water when we are thirsty, and the welcome stretch of our legs as we stroll through a park. It caresses our mind through the lovely colors we see in the fall, and the satisfaction we feel when we see a good movie or solve a mental problem that has been bugging us. But Spirit enters our lives most intimately, gently, and surely through the Virtues of Heart. These virtues are love and love's close relatives, friendship, compassion, and kindness.

Love is in fact the essential nature of Spirit, just as blossoming is the nature of a flower and shining is the nature of the Sun. Take away the blossoming of a flower, and we have some other kind of plant, but not a flower. Take away the shining of the Sun, and we are left with only dead, dark matter. Likewise, if we were to take away love, we would lose Spirit.

Over the centuries, various cultures have conceived of Spirit simply as a powerful, sometimes unpredictable Fundamental Being or Force. But as humankind's understanding has evolved, it has become increasingly clear that Spirit—whether we conceive of it as a personal God, Ultimate Reality, or in some other way—is characterized by profound love.

This explains immediately why two of our dimensions, Spirit and Heart, are so intimately related. In one way of looking at these two dimensions, they are really two aspects of the same thing. Spirit is love, love is

Spirit. It is no wonder then that Spirit is the key to achieving wellness in our social dimension, Heart. And conversely, wellness in Heart, which means to live a life suffused with love, is the key to maximum wellness in our spiritual dimension.

Love and Friendship

When I talk about love, I mean selfless love, what the Ancient Greeks called "arête." This pure form of love is far from the grasping sort of emotion that we sometimes label "love." Selfless love is not grasping at all. On the contrary, it is a deep concern for another being. It is the kind of love most people have for their children and other special people in their lives such as their spouse and parents.

Selfless love is also the basis of true friendship. People often use the term "friends" when they are really talking about casual acquaintances. But we all know that for two people to be real friends, they must have a considerable measure of genuine caring and concern for each other. We may or may not call this "love," but it is clear that it is something similar to love.

To genuinely care for someone, whether family or friends, enhances our wellness in all dimensions, including the physical. This connection to health might surprise some people, but it shouldn't. Scientific research shows that a strong support network of friends and family provides important health benefits. For example, Dr. David Spiegel, a psychiatrist at Stanford University, found that belonging to an emotional support group led to a significant lengthening of life among women with metastatic breast cancer. Other research has shown that people facing serious life issues are much more likely to show resilience and bounce back if they have strong social support. Close relationships in which we feel valued also provide a haven from outside pressures. With family and good friends who care for us, we are able to unwind and "be our self." We can express our thoughts and emotions without worrying about judgment. This results in feelings of belonging, a sense of security, and increased self-esteem, all of which helps counteract that potential killer, stress.

While being cared for by others brings pleasure and promotes peace of mind, caring for someone else can lead to even greater blessings. Loving someone gives us powerful reasons to thrive, benefits our health, and deepens our life satisfaction. Even those who love their pets receive psychological and physiological benefits. Professor Sara Staats at Ohio State University has done research showing that owning pets can help people feel less lonely and depressed and can positively affect their social lives. Another study showed that pet owners had lower blood pressure, triglycerides, and cholesterol levels than non-owners.

Charlene's Experience of Becoming Well by Caring for Others

The boon to wellness that comes from caring for others is illustrated by the experience of Charlene, a forties-something florist whose husband of twenty years, Brian, unexpectedly died of a heart attack.

Charlene and Brian had had a good marriage. But now, since the couple was childless and Charlene's only family lived three thousand miles away, she had no one to care for except her flowers. After Brian's funeral, she became increasingly lonely and depressed. She found much less enjoyment in her business and often closed her store early to go home and go to bed. Her health also started suffering. She caught a couple of bad colds as winter approached, causing her to close her business for days at a time.

Returning home one cold December afternoon, Charlene was surprised to find an elderly woman, dressed only in a nightgown, on her front step. The woman seemed disoriented and muttered that she was waiting for "Diane." Charlene took her inside, got her some blankets, and made her a cup of tea. The woman became more coherent and asked Charlene's pardon for becoming confused and troubling her. She told Charlene her name was Betty, she was 78 years old, and she lived at a nearby elderly residential care facility. She had walked away, wanting to go visit her daughter, Diane. Charlene called the facility, and a worried nurse was soon on her way. In the meantime, Charlene learned a little more about Betty, including that her daughter actually lived in another state and that she received few visitors.

That night, Charlene reflected on how lonely Betty must have been to leave and go looking for her daughter. She decided to visit the woman the next day after work. This she did, and she found Betty to be, despite an occasional memory lapse, an eager and bright conversationalist with wonderful stories to tell about growing up on a farm and being a young mother in the 1950s. What a pity there was no one to listen to those stories, Charlene thought. Afterward, she talked to a nurse and learned that Betty was in the early stages of Alzheimer's. At that point, Charlene made the decision to visit Betty once a week.

Soon, those visits turned into two and three times a week, and then almost every day as Charlene and Betty became close. With someone again to care for, Charlene started feeling more energetic and her enthusiasm for her work returned. She decided she no longer had time for colds because her visits to the residential care home were too important. So if she felt a sore throat coming on, she not only prepared some chicken soup, she made up her mind the cold was not going to get a foothold in her.

As Charlene once again thrived, so did her florist business, and on every visit to Betty, she brought a small bouquet of flowers. Some of the other residents noticed this and asked Charlene if she could bring a flower or two for them too. This she did, and she became known as "The Flower Girl" as she distributed flowers right and left on her visits.

Charlene's experience illustrates the healing power of caring for someone. This is something countless mothers and fathers already know. Parents who have stayed up most of the night with an ill child, then gone to work for a full day, fighting off a cold all the time, know that love can make their immune systems stronger.

Charlene's story also reflects the fact that love and friendship are much more than feelings. They are actions, activities. In Charlene's case, the activity was to take the time and make the effort to visit her new friend. Loving, in short, is doing. Consequently, loving someone or being a caring friend can require work. For one thing, it requires looking past our own desires and viewpoints to see that the other's needs are of equal importance. It demands the ability to empathize with the other person and see things from their point of view. It can take real effort to acknowledge that someone else's perceptions are as valid as our own.

Those who care for no one but themselves may not realize it, but they are confining themselves to a prison constructed by their selfish ego. Locked in their narrow perceptions, needs, and desires, they are unable to see the joy that would come if they were to step out of the bleak, bare walls that surround them into the light of love and true friendship. The only thing fortunate about their situation is that the key to breaking out of their confines is in their grasp at all times. To escape, all they need do is allow themselves to reach out toward someone else with sincere caring. When that happens, love shines purely and the selfish ego all but disappears. In its place, there is a wonderful expansion into the other being. Paradoxically, when we set aside our ego-self by loving another, we make ourselves larger. Loving someone in that way can be profoundly satisfying. For many, it gives life its deepest meaning.

Of course, we all know it can hurt to love someone if the one we love is ill, in danger, or very sad. This is a risk we take in loving. We could insulate ourselves from this potential pain by not caring for anyone, but in the arena of Heart, life would then be empty. Happiness would elude us, for happiness is not simply about enjoying pleasurable activities. A truly happy life has depth and a multitude of facets, with the happiest, most fulfilling life being one with lots of love. And while joy is the gift we receive for loving, pain is the price we must sometimes pay.

Compassion and Kindness

Love goes hand-in-hand with compassion, which is among the greatest of all virtues. In the words of the great philosopher Arthur Schopenhauer, "Compassion is the basis of all morality." Compassion is not pity. It is the recognition of the natural bond between you and someone else who may or may not be having some kind of difficulty. The source of compassion for our fellow humans comes from the realization that no matter what their station in life, they are all blessed people.

This is the message of a traditional Zen story about a young man who wanted to understand what is most worthwhile in life.

To find out, the young man made a long journey to visit a wise monk he had heard about. The monk, who was considered to be a holy man, lived in a cottage high on a mountain. When the young man arrived at the cottage, an old man wielding a broom greeted him at the door.

Taking the old man to be a servant, the young man said, "I came to see the wise holy man."

"Certainly," the old man said and led him inside.

As they walked through the house, the young man's eyes traveled everywhere, eagerly anticipating his meeting with the holy man. Very soon, he was at the back door, whereupon he was escorted outside. He turned to his escort, "But I came to see the holy man!"

"You have," said the old man. "Everyone you may meet in life, even if they appear plain and insignificant—each of them, man, woman, or child—is

holy. If you see people in this way, then whatever question you brought here with you will be answered."

Too many people fail to understand the old monk's lesson. They view one or more segments of society—perhaps people incarcerated, homeless, financially poor, or of a different race—as being somehow "below" them, or even not quite human. That this kind of attitude could still be so widespread is incredible when we all know the horror that occurred in Germany and parts of Eastern Europe in the 1930s and 1940s when an entire racial group was viewed as being of insignificant value compared to the dominant group. Yet millions today carry forward a similar mindset about various groups.

This sad circumstance makes clear the intimate connection between Mind and Heart, for our ability to feel compassion for others (Heart) is inextricably tied to our beliefs about them (Mind). If we believe, for example, that a homeless man or woman pushing a cart full of aluminum cans down the street is unimportant or of no value, then we will feel no compassion for that person. But if we believe that the individual is a blessed child of Spirit, then compassion and a sense of brotherly and sisterly love such as Christ taught will be our natural feeling. And of course, this latter belief is the one that aligns with truth. For there is only one truth here, and it is that every single person in the world is absolutely holy and infinitely valuable. The truth of this statement will already be understood by anyone who has reflected deeply about their beloved child, parent, spouse, or friend.

Like love, compassion is more than a feeling. When put into action, compassion expresses itself as kindness, one of the most beautiful of human qualities. It costs nothing to give someone a smile and a kind greeting, to hold a door open, or to offer a helping hand with a heavy load. There are countless opportunities daily to do so. Taking advantage of those opportunities fosters wellness in all four dimensions:

- Physiologically, kindness is a boon to health by being a form of positivity, which has been linked to a number of health benefits including better immune system functioning, lowered blood pressure, and improved sleep.

- Mentally, kindness creates an optimistic outlook that eases our way through life and makes us feel good about ourselves, both of which have their own physiological advantages.

Kindness Breaks Down Barriers

In my early twenties, I traveled from India to Frankfurt, Germany, for a credentialing exam required to do my residency in the United States. It was my first time away from India. After the exam I had a few days to see West Germany. I had little money, so I traveled mostly by night to save on hotels. I had reached Munich and was strolling through the central city, tightly clutching my small bag with my passport, return ticket for home, and meager funds. Tired from my travel, I sat on a bench to watch a troupe of comedians and became engrossed in the show. When it was over, I rose to continue sightseeing. I walked for ten minutes or so before I discovered, to my horror, that I had left my bag at the street show.

I rushed back but it was nowhere to be found. My heart raced. I asked people nearby if they had seen it. No, they hadn't. I was in a panic, not knowing what to do. Lost among strangers, my eyes fixed on a well-dressed, middle-aged man who looked like he might be a fellow countryman. I approached him and in English said, "Excuse me, are you Indian?"

"No," he replied, "I am Pakistani."

Pakistani! From childhood I had been taught that Pakistanis were my blood enemy. My father had even been stabbed by Pakistanis as they attacked a train he was on. This was the first time I had ever met a Pakistani face to face, and though he didn't look like the brutal ruffian I had always imagined Pakistani men to be, I turned and hurried away.

He caught up with me. "You seem quite stressed," he said. "Can I help you in some way?"

Because I was lost and scared, and because his voice and face seemed so sincere, I blurted out to this total stranger what had happened.

He listened patiently and then said, "Don't worry, I know people here. We will try to find your things. In the meantime, you can come stay with me."

Stay with him? My first thought was that maybe he wanted to lure me to his apartment to beat me up; but reluctantly, I followed him. My qualms were somewhat diminished by meeting his cordial wife and brother, and I shared with them a wonderful dinner. Still, I slept little that night, wondering if I would wake up stabbed, as my father had been.

Next day, sure enough, my bag was somehow located. Extremely relieved, I could now return home.

On the plane, I reflected about my big scare and the fact that a kind man had saved me from what seemed disaster. And by that act of kindness, he had completely shattered my long-held stereotype about Pakistanis. I learned that day that there is no better way to bust through stereotypes and break down barriers than an act of kindness.

- Socially, being kind to others creates an open, pleasing space where people can let their guards down and reach out to one another in friendship. Acts of kindness join people together in a camaraderie that raises both giver and receiver.

- And spiritually, being kind lifts us up and enlarges us just as love and friendship do. Kindness is so beneficial that if you were to perform just five kind acts each day and carry that decision out consistently, it would enrich your life immeasurably.

Overall, compassion and kindness are like love by taking us out of ourselves, enlarging us, and making us noble. The resulting expansion of our ego creates a sense of rightness and well-being that permeates all of our dimensions.

To do good things for others is very natural for most humans, though this capacity may lie hidden if we get lost in the ways of the world. To strengthen it and bring it to fruition, it suffices to begin performing kind actions toward others. As we continue doing so, kindness in time becomes our natural way of acting in the world. Soon, we find ourselves adhering to the wise words of the philosopher Marcus Aurelius: "We ought to do good to others as simply as a horse runs, or a bee makes honey, or a vine bears grapes season after season without thinking of the grapes it has borne." And we learn, personally, the profound truth in the saying of Lao Tzu: "Kindness in words creates confidence. Kindness in thinking creates profundity. Kindness in giving creates love."

Choice and Affirmation

The Virtues of Heart begin with a choice, and for our lives as a whole, it may be our most important one. We can choose to live through ego, competition, grasping, and using others for our own means. Or we can live our lives through love, true friendship, cooperation, compassion, and kindness. Those who choose the first way are often individuals who felt unloved when growing up. Those who choose the second are much more likely to have enjoyed a steady foundation of love as children. Because of this foundation, they feel valuable in themselves and are better able to encompass others in love and kindness.

Since our capacity to love others depends on our ability to love and accept ourselves, it is critical to shower love and affirmation on our children. To affirm our children is not to give them everything they want. Affirmation is consistent with laying down and enforcing sound rules. In fact, setting wise rules is much more consistent with genuine love than an unwise laxity, as long as we also provide our children with reasonable freedom to test themselves in the world. What affirmation means is, simply, to make it perfectly clear to our children at all times that they are infinitely valuable. It is to give them countless hugs and kisses and words that will nurture their strengths and lead them to believe in themselves, their goodness, their abilities, and their future. When we teach our children their own value, we strengthen their capacity to love and we make them ready for the next lesson, which is that we are *all* blessed beings, every single one of us deserving of respect, compassion, and kindness.

Because affirmation is at the very center of love, it is also at the center of love's close relatives: friendship, compassion, and kindness. All of the Virtues of Heart thrive on affirmation. And because love is the essential nature of Spirit, affirmation is also at the center of Spirit. When you consider the other principles of Spirit you are learning in this book, you see again and again that affirmation is at their core: affirmation of ourselves, the other people in our lives, and the world we encounter each day.

It is no exaggeration to say that the Virtues of Heart are the sweetest of human fruits. If we stay within the prison of our ego, if we express only self-centeredness and superficiality in our relations, then we provide only bitter fruit to others—and that is what we will receive from them in return. Worse, our heart will shrivel for being so turned in on itself, and so will our spiritual dimension. But by sharing the Virtues of Heart with others, we nourish and expand both their garden and ours in all dimensions. Love breeds love both in our heart and out in the world. Compassion creates compassion, kindness engenders kindness. What results is a life immersed in Spirit—a vast, heartfelt, loving *Yes* addressed to self, others, and the world.

EXERCISES FOR PRINCIPLE 6: THE VIRTUES OF HEART

Exercise 1: *Greet People with a Smile*

To show kindness and good will often costs only a smile and, especially if you are a man, a nod of the head. This exercise is to be done on a day you are out in public, perhaps shopping or running errands downtown. For every person you pass by, offer a smile and maybe even a kind "Hello" or "How are you?" If the store or sidewalk is too busy, and you can't smile at everyone, pick a few people out and give them a friendly smile as you pass.

Do this for an entire day and note the reactions of the people you walk by. Probably, some recipients of your smiles will give you no reaction, but others will immediately empathize with the kindness you are showing and return the favor. Maybe you will even start a chain reaction as some of those you give smiles to pay it forward to others they pass by.

There are various ways to expand on this experiment of showing a bit of kindness to strangers. Holding a door open for the person behind you is a good way to acknowledge them in a courteous manner. Or when dealing with a salesperson in a store or a teller in a bank, you might notice something about their appearance, such as their clothing or jewelry or hair, and comment favorably on it, saying, for example, "That's a nice pendant" or "I like your tie."

And notice how you yourself feel by extending yourself in kindness to those you meet. Especially when someone returns your smile, isn't that a nice pick-me-up? At the end of the day, reflect on what you have been doing and what a more pleasant world it would be if everyone behaved the same way, smiling at strangers, holding doors open, finding something to say that will show your appreciation of the reality and goodness of another person.

Now extend your experiment to the next day, and the next, and the next . . .

Exercise 2: *Care for Others by Doing Something Unexpected*

We all know that special days are set aside for showing others we care about them. Think of Valentine's Day, Christmas, birthdays, and anniversaries. But how about all the rest of the days of the year? Of course we often show our caring for others daily by working to earn a paycheck, cooking and cleaning, and being there to listen to them about whatever their concerns may be. But as for giving the other people in our lives a little special recognition, why should we restrict ourselves to only a few days in the year?

This exercise is about occasionally doing something special and unexpected for those you love to show them how special you think they are. Here are five ways to surprise them on some otherwise ordinary (of course no day is really ordinary) Tuesday in March or Thursday in October. Choose a few of these ways of demonstrating your feelings and just do them. Even better, choose all of the ways.

1. For your spouse or sweetheart, locate a greeting card that speaks of your love for them not just on Valentine's Day but on some random day. Place it beside their plate or bowl before they sit down for breakfast, or present the card the next time you see them, perhaps along with a single rose.

2. This same kind of thing can be done for a child, parent, or friend by locating an appropriate card that tells of your affection and surprising them with it. You know it's a good idea, a win-win initiative.

3. Think hard about some gift that someone you care about would really like to receive. Then don't wait for Christmas or a birthday to get it for them. Go out today, buy the item, wrap it up to make it even more special, and watch their eyes light up when you surprise them "for no reason." Of course, you know the reason: because you love them.

4. What could you do today to lighten the daily responsibilities of your spouse, parent, or friend? What chore that is usually theirs and not yours would allow them a little more leisure time if you were to take it on yourself for at least one day? Washing the dishes? Raking the lawn? Watching your friend's baby so she can go to the movie with her husband? Figure out what chore you can take on for someone you care about and then give them this very thoughtful present from your heart.

5. How long has it been since you've done something special with your spouse, kids, or friend? How long since you and your spouse have been out to dinner, how long since you've taken the kids to the zoo or the entire family on a picnic? And how long since you've invited your friend to join you at whatever game is in town? Why not do it today, tomorrow, or this weekend? Surprise your spouse with dinner out (let him or her choose the restaurant); surprise the kids with a day at the water park; surprise your friend by inviting him or her for a hike or a walk in the park.

You get the idea. It doesn't take a lot to show someone how special they are to you.

✿

Harmony

Live in Unity and Balance

*"Happiness is when what you think, what you say,
and what you do are in harmony."*
Mahatma Ghandi
quoted in *Humor, Play, and Laughter* by J.A. Michelli

From the beginning of time, Spirit has infused all of Reality with blessed harmony. When we look up to the sky on a clear, moonless night, the array of light spread out above us may appear jumbled and random. But giant telescopes tell us a different story. Some of the pinpoints of light we see are immense galaxies of stars spinning slowly in beautiful spirals. Most are individual stars burning with a dynamic internal balance that enables them to pour forth light for eons. A few are planets swinging in regular, measured arcs around our Sun. At the grandest level, balance, order, and harmonious movement are signature qualities of the universe.

Here on Earth, too, harmony is the hallmark of nature. The beautiful design of an eagle's wings, the ceaseless back and forth of the moonstruck tides, the perfect symmetry of a single snowflake. Everywhere we look we see order and balance. Where harmony exists, there is always a rhythm, a cycle of events, shapes, sounds, or colors that occur with regularity. We see this in the passage of the four seasons with its rhythm of growth, maturity, decay, and rebirth. Nature's yearly harmony happens as each season plays its proper part in the whole. Without the snows of winter and the rains of spring, there can be no growth in summer, no harvest in fall. In turn, the decaying leaves of fall and winter help nourish the rebirth that comes with spring.

Because we are nature's offspring, harmony also permeates our own existence—or at least it should. Each dimension of our lives has its own distinctive ways of being in tune. When we lack wellness in one of our dimensions, it is harmony that we lack. To be totally well is to be in harmony with ourselves, other people, nature, and Spirit.

To understand harmony, we can begin with the fact that everything, living or inanimate, consists of parts. Harmony occurs when those parts work together in unison, each one doing its particular job for the benefit of the subject's overall structure. Where harmony does not exist in our lives, we find disorder and sometimes chaos. Where it does exist, our various aspects—physical, mental, social, and spiritual—function properly and are at equilibrium, though often a very dynamic equilibrium.

Harmony of Body

Harmony begins with our bodies, which are extremely complex systems whose rhythms are many. Each bodily subsystem, cardiovascular, digestive, nervous, and others, is composed of numerous parts that work together to perform crucial physiological functions. And since these subsystems overlap and affect each other, they all must work together in harmony if our body is to be in balance. When things go wrong, for example when a virus enters a person's body, the immune system goes to work. If the immune defense is strong, it may successfully fight off the invader. If not, the person's bodily systems may become unbalanced and disordered, jeopardizing his or her health.

But bodily harmony is not just about the interior of our body. It is also about the interaction of our physical subsystems with the external world. We now understand the importance of establishing a harmonious relation between ourselves and the world outside. The sunshine that falls on our skin, the cereal we eat in the morning, the air we take into our lungs, these all become part of our physical self. Our body is actually an extension of the external world, and if we allow it to fall out of harmony with that world, our physical health suffers. Nature, as we have learned, is a double-edged sword. The food, liquid, air, and other substances we ingest are capable of strengthening our bodily systems, or weakening them. Physical wellness, then, is about harmonizing our bodily needs and functions with what we take in from the outside world.

Harmony of Mind

Since wellness spans all of our dimensions, we must seek more than just bodily harmony. For total wellness all four dimensions must be in balance in themselves and with each other. This is very clear in the case of our mental life. Wellness of Mind implies several kinds of harmony. First, it means being at peace with the world. We saw in the discussion about the Principle of Calmness how chronic stress caused by worry and anxiety can make our hormones run wild. Lack of mental harmony leads to physical imbalances, impedes our social life, and leads us away from spiritual principles that foster wellness. This is why finding effective ways to overcome stress leads to greater harmony in all aspects of our lives.

Harmony can also elude us mentally when our desire to lead a healthful life contradicts a craving for a harmful substance or behavior, such as tobacco, alcohol, drugs, or gambling. These cravings can easily become addictions, some so strong they may require withdrawal to a hospital-like setting. I understand how hard it is to fight such addictions, because I have been there, with both alcohol and cigarettes. I know how obsessive cravings can disrupt lives, curtail harmony in many ways, and undermine wellness. Addictions like these are primarily medical issues, and for anyone reading this who has a harmful substance or behavioral addiction, I highly recommend discussing your situation thoroughly with your physician. The medical sciences have made some important breakthroughs in treating various addictions, for instance smoking, and you need to be aware of the best tools available to restore balance and harmony.

There are many other instances in which we have conflicting desires, but they are usually relatively mild. Common examples are the dieter tempted to order a hamburger and fries instead of a Cobb salad, the homeowner who wants to go window shopping instead of cleaning the house, and the aspiring doctor who yearns to take a night off to watch TV instead of cracking the books. We all give in to such common temptations once in a while, but that's not necessarily a bad thing. To occasionally give ourselves a certain degree of slack as we work toward our goals may be necessary for our overall harmony and wellness. If it becomes too much slack, however, we may find ourselves in a position similar to that of Beth, a college sophomore who was majoring in pre-Med.

How Beth Gave in to Temptation

Beth was a busy student who took part in various campus activities, studied hard, and prided herself on getting straight A's in her classes. Then a friend introduced her to online social networking sites, and she immediately got hooked. She began spending hours every evening on the Internet, socializing and playing games, which left much less time for her school work. Her studies began suffering, and her offline social life became almost nonexistent. At the same time, her weight started ballooning because she felt she no longer had time for her evening workout at the gym. She was also snacking more as she stayed up late trying to keep up with her studies. As the days rolled by, Beth felt her life becoming increasingly disordered as she fought against her urges to have "fun" online—but without success. When her next grade report came out and she received two B's and three C's she knew she had to make some changes. But after agonizing for weeks, she still couldn't find the will to substantially reduce the time she spent online. For a while she contemplated dropping out of college, but she decided to continue, even in the face of her continuing addiction. As a result, she went from being an exceptional student to settling for mediocre achievement and so-so grades, a pattern that would eventually make it difficult for her to be accepted into a good medical school.

Beth's internal conflicts may not have risen to the urgency of a substance addiction, but they were still quite destructive of her mental harmony, not to mention her plans for her future. While she was socializing online, she may have been able to block out the conflict. But as soon as she returned to her collegiate world, it was there in full force, badgering her. Her mental conflict also disrupted the physical and social dimensions of her life.

How we handle the various temptations that may lead us away from where we want most to go in our lives can affect our inner harmony, our wellness, and of course how successful we are in our endeavors. It takes practical wisdom to know how to balance our desires so they work together harmoniously. Beth may have possessed this practical wisdom in other aspects of her life, but it failed her when it came to balancing her craving for easy entertainment with her desire to do well in her studies and eventually enroll in medical school.

Self-Knowledge

Our best strategy for gaining the practical wisdom we need to deal with conflicting desires is to maximize our self-knowledge. When we fall prey to behaviors we know are self-destructive, it is usually because we are not clear about who we are and what we want. We lose inner harmony as we fight against ourselves, sabotaging our own nature because we do not really know what it is. Unfortunately, to understand ourselves at a deep level can be difficult these days. It would seem that understanding who we are, where we want to go, and who we want to become would be easier than ever at this time in history when a world of information in the form of books, websites, and other media is at our fingertips. But it is probably more difficult today than ever before to gain true and deep knowledge of ourselves. This is because, due to modern technology, we are almost constantly bombarded by advertisements, political messages, and societal expectations that tell us what we should believe, look like, hope for, and pursue in our lives. A glut of directives washes over us from every direction, flooding us with thousands of contradictory messages announcing what others think we should do and be. To fight our way out of this constant noise, to go deep inside and understand clearly who we are and truly want to be in the future, can be a formidable job. Yet we must perform that job if we are to achieve maximum harmony in our lives.

Self-knowledge begins with the kind of understanding I talked about in my discussion of the Principle of Dharma—to recognize our most fundamental interests and talents so that we can have a clear idea of our natural road in life, our dharma road. Part of what led Beth to neglect her studies may have been that she was not sure she wanted to be a doctor. She needed to confront the question of how much she actually wanted to fulfill that goal, and demand honest answers from herself. If she had done so, she might have discovered she was traveling down the wrong road and that being a physician was not really what she wanted to do with her life. On the other hand, she might have realized more clearly than ever that becoming a medical doctor was the career she aspired to more than any other, a realization that would have helped her limit her online socializing. Clearly understanding the goals that have the greatest meaning for us, the ones we want most to achieve, helps keep us moving strongly along the path to achieving those goals.

Sometimes, in seeking self-knowledge, we may discover that we have not been true to ourselves. The ways in which our parents, friends, associates, or society itself have defined us may not correspond to the person we feel we actually are. This can cause a deep disharmony in not only our mental, but also our social and spiritual dimensions. An example is the

Following Your Dharma Road Prevents Addictions

Self-knowledge includes knowing your purpose in life. It is difficult for addictions, whether to alcohol, drugs, gambling, or something else, to take root if you feel yourself making progress toward fulfilling your life's purpose. When you are on your dharma road, you feel happy just being on your way. You have no time or inclination for addictive behavior that might become an obstacle or even lead you off that road.

Conversely, if you have no purpose that beckons you, then it is easier to become lost on byways that can turn into addictions.

There was a time when I flirted too closely with several addictions, including to alcohol and status-seeking. I know now that this was partly due to my not having discovered my true purpose in life. As I became increasingly certain that my proper role is to be a healer not just of the body but of the mind, heart, and spirit, there was no longer any space for addictions to take hold. It is often confusion about what we want to achieve in our lives that constitutes the soil in which addictions can take root. By becoming clear on our dharma road and on what has greatest meaning in our life, that soil disappears.

Today I am very happy to say that my flirtation with addictions has given way to the guidance of Loving Spirit, and a desire to do the best I can to create hope, harmony, and healing in the world.

fact that in this society, boys and girls are typically expected to behave in certain ways. If they do not, they are castigated or even ostracized by their peers, and often criticized by their elders. This circumstance is unfortunate for the nonaggressive boy who does not like to play physical games or with toy guns, but who instead demonstrates an artistic and sensitive nature. It is also unfortunate for the girl who does not like to play with dolls or dress up but would rather climb a tree or play football with the boys. Though male and female stereotypes may not be as strong as they were a few decades ago, they are often still powerful enough to drive an individual away from his or her own nature. This can create a powerful inner discord in the child and in the adult the child becomes. It is a disharmony that can only be resolved when the person understands and embraces his or her true nature. Though we are in many ways the products of society, who we are most authentically must be defined primarily by what is inside us, not by what others expect or demand.

Harmony of Heart and Spirit

Self-knowledge is also about understanding what values we hold most dear. When we ask ourselves about our values, it helps to think in terms of the traditional virtues. Of these, there are two main kinds. The first consists of the *Virtues of the Heart* we discussed earlier: love, friendship, compassion, and kindness. The second kind I call *Virtues of Character.* Examples are honesty, fidelity, courage, gentleness, and humility. These are values that almost all people uphold, if not in their actions, at least in their words and aspirations. Virtually all of us, when we search ourselves deeply, will find that we believe in the value of courage, honesty, and the other Virtues of Character. We also often feel that moments when our actions are guided by such values are among the finest moments of our lives.

To reflect on the Virtues of Heart and Character, and to ask which of them we want to exhibit in our lives, can go a long way toward clarifying what we stand for and who we want to be. This, in turn, can help us withstand temptations that might take us away from those values. For example, a husband's clear realization that fidelity to his wife is of paramount importance to him can help him turn away from any temptation to step outside that marriage. And an expectant mother who smokes but who comes to a clear, explicit understanding that preserving the health of her unborn child is of highest value to her will be very strongly motivated to give up her smoking habit.

One reason almost all of us admire and want to posses the Virtues of Character is that they are spiritual values. Recall that we learned that the Virtues of Heart are spiritual values because the essence of Spirit is love. But if this is true, the Virtues of Character must also be spiritual values, because truly loving someone, whether our spouse, child, relative, or friend, requires us to be ready at all times to display the virtues of honesty, fidelity, courage, and gentleness. Indeed, how could we possibly love someone without being ready to exercise those qualities when needed? And when we embrace those indispensable values, we immediately create greater harmony in our lives.

Here, as everywhere, harmony is the reflection of Spirit. Because of this, harmony enters our lives most fully when we allow our spiritual dimension to flourish. By doing so, we are able to create an all-embracing context in which we can make sense of our lives. My earlier description of Emily is a wonderful example of this. Recall that Emily was feeling intense disharmony in her life as her wellness in Body, Mind, and Heart declined. The questions about life that were plaguing her, causing her to lose sleep, were valid ones: "Why am I working so hard? What is the purpose of my life? Is it just all about money?" We all should be asking such questions. But we must understand that the only way we will find answers to them is through our spiritual dimension. This is what Emily learned. When she began embracing her spirituality, she was able to view her life in the light of broad principles of Spirit. Allowing her spiritual aspect to have its say, she arrived at her three-part conclusion: the purpose of her life was simply to love and help provide for her family; try to be a strong, compassionate businessperson; and enjoy each day. Others who seek the purpose or meaning of their lives may come to different conclusions. But like Emily, they will discover that asking and answering the "big" questions sets them on the road to greater harmony in their lives.

We also allow our spiritual dimension to flourish by opening ourselves to the Virtues of Heart. Just as we are intimately connected to the physical world surrounding us, we are continuous with our fellow humans. We are not meant to isolate ourselves so that all of our thoughts and emotions are focused on the needs and desires of our selfish ego. We are social beings, and to be social means more than to socialize. It means to reach out in respect, compassion, kindness, and genuine caring to our family, friends, and neighbors. To say this creates harmony in our lives is an understatement. The most important part of living a harmonious life is to love others and to feel their love, caring, and friendship in return.

In sum, there are four main strategies to maximize harmony in the four dimensions of our lives. The first strategy is to promote bodily harmony by balancing inner nature with outer nature. It is to eat, drink, and breathe in only what keeps our bodily systems in their natural and proper dynamic balance.

The second and third strategies are meant to promote mental harmony. The second is to calm the turbulence caused by stress. The third is to discover our deepest authentic self. To do this, we must understand what projects and goals will give our lives their greatest meaning. We must also do our best to clarify what we want to stand for in our lives—our values. Then we must let all this knowledge help us balance our various desires harmoniously and guide us along our dharma road.

The fourth strategy is to promote inner harmony by allowing our spiritual dimension to bear fruit. This is a powerful strategy because ultimately, Spirit is the source of all harmony and wellness. To open our spiritual dimension fully, we must cling to the Virtues of Heart and Character. To live in harmony is to live in love and kindness, camaraderie and compassion. It is also to express, in our actions toward ourselves and others, fidelity, honesty, and the other Virtues of Character. By embracing these spiritual values, we create a comprehensive context that brings deep meaning to our daily actions and promotes harmony in all aspects of life.

EXERCISES FOR PRINCIPLE 7: HARMONY

Exercise 1: *Understand Bodily Harmony*

For the purposes of this exercise we can name ten major bodily systems that make up your physiology. These systems are the cardiovascular, digestive, respiratory, musculoskeletal, nervous, urinary, immune, reproductive, integumentary (skin), and endocrine (glandular) systems.

For the exercise itself, your goal is to consider some or all of the ten common substances and bodily inputs listed below and learn which of the ten bodily systems each one affects and how. Is the effect negative or positive? Or does negativity or positivity depend on how much you ingest or breathe in? Record what you learn in a notebook or a computer file. And don't assume that an item affects only one or two systems, because some affect more systems than is immediately obvious. This exercise will require some research skills and may require several hours of your time, but if you complete the exercise for each of the items listed, you will gain some important understandings of how your bodily systems behave given the effects of these inputs.

Here is the list of bodily inputs, with space for you to name all of the bodily systems listed above that they each affect.

Salt _____

_____

Sugar _____

_____

Cigarette smoke _____

_____

Alcohol _____

_____

Fish oil _____

_____

Carrots _____

_____

Saturated fats _____

_____

Stress _____

_____

Kind acts directed at you _____

_____

Kind acts performed by you _____

_____

Exercise 2: *Discover Where You Stand Among the Virtues of Heart and Character*

As we have learned above (see Make Thinking Your Powerful Ally), each of us can be defined in many different ways at any one time. One way we define ourselves, if only implicitly, is through the values we adhere to. These definitions tend to describe us on a deep level. Of course, our values may change over a lifetime, but the changes are usually gradual. We are unlikely to wake up some morning and in our actions suddenly turn our back on whatever values have guided us for the last ten or twenty years. But even though values tend to define us on a deep level, it would be difficult for many people to state clearly, even if pressed, what values guide them. In this way, their explicit self-knowledge is deficient.

This exercise is designed to encourage you to think explicitly about your values, and in particular, the Virtues of Heart and Character. For the purposes of this exercise, let's consider these values to be the following:

Fidelity	Love	Courage
Compassion	Gentleness	Honesty
Tolerance	Good Humor	Self-control
Good judgment	Gratitude	Kindness

The first step in this exercise is to number these values from 1 to 12, with 1 meaning you feel the value is the most important in your life, and 12 meaning the value that is the least important. Use a pencil in case you change your mind about their proper order part way through.

The second step is to go deeper in your thinking about each of these values. You may do this by setting aside an hour or two to consider each of these values in turn, one by one, for five to ten minutes. For each one, ask yourself and answer three sets of questions:

- What does having this value entail? To what degree does this value guide my life? Is it important to me, or does it matter only moderately, slightly, or not at all?

- What are one or two recent instances when I demonstrated this value by my actions? What was the outcome? Are there any instances in which I violated this value through my actions? If so, what was the outcome, and how do I feel about those instances now?

- How much do I want to be someone who adheres to this value in the future? To what extent do I want others to adhere to this value in their dealings with me?

The third step in the exercise is to again number the values from 1 to 12 after having thought about them and their place in your life at some depth. Have any risen in your estimation? Is it more difficult to decide which are the most important values than it was in the first step? Here are the values again for you to again number if the order of what you consider most important in your life has changed.

Fidelity	Love	Courage
Compassion	Gentleness	Honesty
Tolerance	Good Humor	Self-control
Good judgment	Gratitude	Kindness

∽

Seva

Accept the Gift of Selfless Service

"Don't look for big things,
just do small things with great love."
Mother Teresa
quoted in *Mother Teresa: Come Be My Light*
by B. Kolodiejchuk

What often blocks us from realizing we are children of Spirit is our selfish ego. The ego is a product of evolution. For early humans, every day was a battle for survival in a hard world. Primitive men and women had to focus on their personal well-being almost constantly. Eyes, ears, and noses had to be on guard to avoid deadly dangers that might be lurking behind any bush or tree. Social life was dominated by competition to gain the most valuable resources, such as the biggest portions of whatever food was available, the sharpest pieces of stone for spearheads, the most goats or chickens, the brightest body ornamentation. Over eons, this deep-seated concern for survival, possessions, and prestige evolved into our self-centered ego.

Today, some people in the world continue to deal with very difficult and dangerous circumstances. But most of us do not—at least not nearly to the degree that was true for primitive humans. Yet even in these less risky times, our ego is typically on duty at every moment as if we were still back on the savannah, focusing on our survival and trying to surpass our neighbors any way we can.

The selfish ego we have inherited from our dangerous and competitive past is at the opposite pole from Spirit. The selfish ego is about ME, while Spirit is about US. The selfish ego is grasping and greedy, while Spirit is kind and giving. The selfish ego is inward looking and restricted, while Spirit is outgoing, expansive, and in fact infinite.

So are we simply stuck with our self-centered, grasping ego? Or is there another type of ego that is possible for humans? What if we could bypass the effects of thousands of years of competing with others and discover within ourselves an ego that goes hand-in-hand with Spirit? Is that possible?

The Spiritual Ego

There is, indeed, a type of ego that is the opposite of the selfish version. Instead of constantly looking inward, it looks outward toward others. Instead of being grasping, it is open and giving. Instead of being only about ME, it holds out a hand to others. It is, simply, our ego as infused and fed by Spirit. In a word, it is our *spiritual ego.*

Some would claim that the idea of a spiritual ego is a contradiction in terms. They might say that by its nature, the ego is always self-focused and egotistical. But this is a misunderstanding based on a narrow understanding of what an ego is. Most basically, the word "ego" simply means the self. My ego is my individual *self.* Yours is your individual self. And there is no reason to think that the self must always be totally focused on its own desires and needs. On the contrary, it can be directed outward toward other people and the natural world.

Our spiritual ego is as much as product of evolution as our selfish ego. Certainly, primitive humans competed with one another in many ways, but they also had to cooperate and help each other in order to survive. As a result, along with the self-seeking aspect of the ego, there evolved a more cooperative, outward-looking, other-person-directed side. This outer-directed aspect is our spiritual ego.

Almost all of us possess this kind of ego at least some of the time. For instance, we experience ourselves as having a spiritual ego when we look at a sleeping baby and are flooded with a sense of wanting to protect the child. We experience our spiritual ego when we yearn to comfort a friend who is going through a difficult time. We experience our spiritual ego when we look at a beautiful sunset and feel our mind expanding into the sky. At these times, our thoughts and emotions are selfless. They are not about Me, but about the welfare of someone else or the pure beauty of what we observe. And this version of our ego is not at the opposite pole from Spirit. On the contrary, it is intimately intertwined with Spirit. It is, in fact, Spirit working within us, transcending our selfish desires, breaking down the barriers between self and others, and drawing us closer to our fellow humans and the rest of the natural world.

What results from this infusion of Spirit is an enlargement of the ego. This enlargement consists of a wonderful expansion of the self so that it includes other people. To understand what I mean, consider your experience when you feel yourself caring for the well-being of your child, parent, spouse, or friend. Is it not true that when you care deeply, you feel as if the other person is somehow a part of you? And in fact they are, for when you truly care for someone else, the boundaries of your self expand to take in the other person. Not physically, of course, but mentally and spiritually, in your thoughts and emotions. When that happens, our ego also becomes mentally and spiritually stronger and more confident than it ever is in selfish mode. When we pursue objectives for only selfish reasons, we are actually weaker in ourselves than when our pursuits are directed toward the well-being of others.

We began discovering some of this when we talked about how Spirit reveals itself through the Virtues of Heart. We learned that when we practice love and the other virtues, we rise above our self-centered concerns and nurture our larger self. We also learned that love is not just a feeling. It is an activity. To love someone requires putting forth effort when effort is needed by that someone. The same goes for friendship, compassion, and kindness. If these are to be genuine emotions, and not mere transitory feelings, then they must lead us into action. In particular, if we want our spiritual ego to thrive and flourish to its maximum extent, we must understand and practice something called *Seva*.

Seva

Seva is a Sanskrit word that is similar in meaning to the English word "altruism." Seva means *selfless service.* The essence of Seva is to perform actions not for the sake of ourselves, but for others. Seva consists of both an attitude and a way of acting. The attitude is one of respect and concern for the well-being of other people. That attitude gives rise to Seva as a natural way of acting toward others, which is to understand their legitimate needs and help fulfill those needs with no expectation of return.

Seva occurs when a dentist gives part of his or her professional time, for no charge, to treat the dental problems of needy children. It occurs when a practicing physician decides to join a humanitarian group such as Doctors without Borders in order to help stem disease in a poverty-stricken country. Seva occurs when a church group travels to an earthquake-ravaged region in order to set up temporary shelters for the victims of the disaster.

But we need not be a dentist, a doctor, or church member to practice Seva. Selfless service happens whenever we give part of our time and effort to the well-being of others. It could be helping to teach an adult to read or to deliver food in a nutritional program for elderly people living at home. It could be helping fellow townspeople clean up after a flood or working with a group to create a hiking trail so others can enjoy an outdoor area. There are thousands of worthwhile projects awaiting our efforts.

The Spiritual Principle of Seva is simply this:

> *Give of yourself for the well-being of others,*
> *and let the giving be your only reward.*

Seva is an ancient concept. Virtually every major religion includes Seva as a major part of its beliefs. In Christianity, for example, we find many admonitions similar to the biblical directive in Philippians 2.3-4: "Let each of you look not only to his own interests, but also to the interests of others."

In Hinduism, the *Bhagavad Gita* says, in 3.10-26, "Strive constantly to serve the welfare of the world; by devotion to selfless work, one attains the supreme goal in life. Do your work with the welfare of others always in mind."

In Taoism, the *Tao Te Ching* includes the following passage:

"The sage does not accumulate for himself.

The more he uses for others, the more he has himself.

The more he gives to others, the more he possesses of his own.

The Way of Heaven is to benefit others and not to injure.

The Way of the sage is to act but not to compete." (81)

In these and other religious traditions, the idea of selfless service appears repeatedly as a way to become closer to God or Spirit. This is understandable since Spirit emphasizes the unity that is present in the millions of diverse individuals that we humans are. And there is no better way for each of us to promote unity than through selfless service to others.

Selfless service is also a very familiar concept in our secular culture. An excellent example is the well-known classic movie, *It's a Wonderful Life*. The movie tells the story of George Bailey, who sacrificed his powerful desire to see the world in order to stay home and extend himself for the sake of his town and its people. By doing so, he bettered their lives in many ways, which acted as a stabilizing force on the town. George was unaware of the immensely beneficial results of his actions until he had the opportunity to see how the town would have deteriorated if he had never been born. The idea of selfless service also permeates our society in the form of well-known heroes such as Florence Nightingale, Mahatma Gandhi, Martin Luther King, Jr., and Mother Teresa, all of whom served the cause of individuals or groups of people with no thought of reward.

Two Keys to Seva

There are two essential keys to the practice of true Seva. One is that Seva requires us to put forth personal effort. Giving money to a cause is good, but it is not enough. Our most precious assets are our time and energy, our intelligence and sweat. When we devote our personal efforts to a worthwhile cause that we believe in, we are practicing genuine Seva.

Unfortunately, some never take the first step toward selfless service because they think they have no time to spare. But no matter how busy we may be in our lives, there is almost always at least a few hours a week that we can spend for the sake of others. In many cases, just a small amount of time can be of great value to someone in need of help. This is well illustrated by what an office worker named Thomas learned soon after he began volunteering to help cook and serve meals at a homeless shelter.

Thomas's Lesson about the Practice of Seva

Thomas knew he was doing a good thing by helping two nights a week at the shelter, and he was glad to do it. But after he had volunteered for three months, he became convinced that his efforts had no long-range effect on the people he served. That was because every time he was there, he seemed to see the same faces at the table, mostly men but also a few women. He didn't think much about the particular circumstances that might have led those individuals to be without a home, but the one thing that seemed clear to him was that once they were on the street, they stayed there.

One evening as Thomas and Jeff, the manager of the shelter, were cleaning up after dinner, Thomas mentioned that he sometimes felt he was doing very little for the homeless people by helping serve them dinner. "It's just one meal," he said, "and they need a lot more than that to get back on their feet."

Jeff looked at Thomas in a puzzled way. "Do you really think a hot meal means that little to these folks? Actually, Thomas, you are doing much more good here than you realize."

"How can you say that?" Thomas replied. "The clientele here never changes. These are obviously chronic homeless people."

"That may be true for some, but certainly not all," Jeff replied. "You've been volunteering here for three months. I've been managing this place for ten years. And I have seen many success stories over that time. Yes, when people become homeless, it often takes months for them to get enough money together to find their own place to live. But many manage to do just that. Some of the faces you saw here tonight will be out looking for a job tomorrow—and the next day and the next. And can you imagine the difference between going out into the world to look for work having had a decent meal the night before and going out hungry?"

When Thomas shrugged, Jeff laughed and said, "Thomas, do you know that I myself was homeless at one time, before I was married? I had lost my job because of a factory shutdown, and there was no other work available. I was soon out on the street. Every night I came to a place like this for a meal. And that meal was the only thing that kept me going as I pounded the streets looking for a job. Finally, after almost six months, I got a job and started pulling myself back up. Don't think for one moment that a hot meal can't make a huge difference in a person's energy and attitude, because it can. You may not know who you are helping to get back on their feet here each evening, but you can bet you are aiding some of those folks in a big way."

From his conversation with Jeff, Thomas learned that there are times and situations when just a little help can be a key to greatly improving a person's life. Not knowing for sure how much difference we are making should never be used as a basis for withholding our efforts.

Another reason some people never step into Seva is because they feel they have nothing to offer. But that is never true. What each of us can contribute to the world is our individual self: our personality, our interactions with others, what we have experienced, what we have learned. We all have something we are good at, talents that can go toward helping others meet whatever challenges they may face or making the world a more enjoyable and rewarding place for others. If it is unclear just how and where to volunteer your efforts for the sake of others, a little research will likely uncover many possibilities. Probably in your own community, there are schools, hospitals, hospices, parks, senior citizen centers, and other organizations that welcome volunteers for different kinds of roles. Don't wait until you feel you are able to do something "big," but rather follow the words of President Theodore Roosevelt: "Do what you can, with what you have, where you are." The first exercise at the end of this chapter will help you identify organizations that could use your services, along with identifying the skills, abilities, knowledge, and experience that are unique to you and that you could bring to a volunteer effort.

The second key to the practice of genuine Seva is to perform our service for others simply for their sake, not for some extrinsic reward. Unfortunately, there is an argument that has been floating around for some years that humans never do anything for the sake of others. Supposedly, since doing altruistic acts makes the actor feel good, the acts are, at root, not altruistic at all, but selfish. This is not only a sad argument, it is a poor one. If Thomas feels good about cooking and serving dinner for homeless people, that does not make him selfish. It makes him into a man who at least sometimes thinks of the welfare of others and does something about it. To claim people are selfish if they enjoy helping others is a gross misuse of the term "selfish."

The Many Rewards of Seva

Even though genuine acts of Seva are never done for a reward, the marvelous fact is that doing things for others promotes wellness in all dimensions. Physiologically, there is increasing scientific evidence that helping others has important benefits to our physical health. This includes a decade-long study of 2,700 men in Michigan that found a significantly lower death rate among those who did regular volunteer work. Another study of over 50,000 elderly people in California found that those who volunteered for two or more organizations had significantly lower mortality than those who did not volunteer. In addition, Duke University Medical Center researchers discovered that recovering heart patients who volunteered to visit current heart patients had a sixty percent faster recovery rate than those who did not volunteer. Selflessly helping others has also been found to have a calming influence on the emotions, thereby combating stress. Research has also shown that helping others promotes psychological well-being. One study found that hospital patients and their family members who volunteered to support other patients had increased emotional wellness. Another study showed that multiple sclerosis (MS) patients who gave peer support to other MS patients increased their self-esteem, self-awareness, confidence, and daily functioning. Researchers at the University of Massachusetts Medical School state that when volunteers focus on others, this combats the self-focused character of anxiety and depression.

Practicing Seva promotes mental health because it connects us to something valuable outside us. When we contribute, we typically get back much more emotionally than we give, in the form of feeling that we are part of a worthwhile project. When we give sincerely of ourselves, the resulting satisfaction far outweighs the time required. We quickly find that the time we spend in volunteering is precious in itself, and very likely to be among our most valuable and fulfilling moments.

Selflessly doing for others also has other mental and emotional benefits by energizing our lives beyond our volunteer role. It increases our self-esteem, broadens our perspectives, and sharpens our thinking, all of which better enables us to deal with whatever comes our way. In addition, when we are beset by problems in our own lives, there is often no better way to put those problems in perspective than to focus on the well-being of others. Recall the experience of Charlene, who had lost not only her husband, but her enjoyment of life. She was despondent until she decided to start visiting her new friend Betty, who had few visitors otherwise. There is no doubt that her visits were of great value to Betty and perhaps even to other elderly residents of the facility, but the greatest value was enjoyed by Charlene herself, as she found her attitude toward life changing dramatically.

Seva promotes wellness most obviously in our social dimension—Heart. When we work selflessly for the well-being of others, their needs

By Serving You, I Serve Myself

These words—"By serving you, I serve myself"—attributed to Lao Tzu, are worth pondering.

For one thing, there are the medical benefits that one receives from giving, including the reduction of stress hormones such as cortisol and epinephrine, the increases in good hormones such as DHEA and prolactine, and other health benefits.

And there is the satisfaction felt from reaching out to others to benefit them in some way. Knowing that our connecting to others is motivated solely by concern for their well being can bring a priceless and pure sense of joy.

Not long ago, I was in a grocery line and the man ahead of me was searching his pockets for change, as he was short of money for an item. He was about to return the item when I asked the cashier to put the price of it on my bill. The man was very thankful. And I noticed that I too felt thankful that I had been given the opportunity to help the man out in this small way. I like to think that the man will remember the encounter, and that at some point in the future he will pay it forward by helping someone else who is in a grocery line short on money or who is in some other predicament.

And what did this act require of me? A mere dollar or so. What a small price to pay to connect on a compassionate and understanding level with another human being!

and aspirations become partly our own. Our dimension of Heart prospers as we feel ourselves joined, at least temporarily, to their lives. And because Heart is the soul of Spirit, our spiritual wellness soars as we are infused with new meaning.

From all of this, it becomes abundantly clear that those who practice Seva, though they seek no reward, are often the ones who receive the greatest gifts from their efforts. I hope that one of those blessed people is, or soon will be, you.

EXERCISES FOR PRINCIPLE 8: SEVA

Exercise 1: *Six Steps to Volunteering for a Worthy Cause*

As you learned above, one of the essential characteristics of practicing Seva is that it goes beyond contributing money to a worthwhile cause or organization. Practicing Seva requires putting your energy, knowledge, and experience to work for others. One great way to do this is to volunteer some time each week to a worthwhile cause or organization.

Maybe you are already someone who is quick to lend a helping hand to others through volunteering for a social agency or other organization. If so, congratulations and thank you. But if you are slow to volunteer or feel your efforts in this direction could be improved, and especially if you are not already aware of some volunteer activity that might match your abilities and schedule, this exercise is for you. The exercise is to follow a practical six-step process that can lead you to become a volunteer. Here are the six steps:

Step 1. Using the Internet, newspaper, friends, and whatever other resources you can access, learn which social agencies and organizations in your area may have needs for volunteer support. Make a list of these organizations, their missions and responsibilities, and the locations of their local headquarters.

Step 2. Now make a list of whatever talents, skills, interests, education, attitude, and experience you have that might be valuable to one or more of these organizations. You don't have to uncover some esoteric skills or knowledge that no one else has. Just list the things you know how to do. Do you drive? That's a skill. Do you read? That's a skill too. And there are organizations that can make good use of one or both of them. Here are some other skills and qualities that come to mind: good with children, patient, know a foreign language, strong, good with numbers, cheerful, proficient cook, own a pickup. Any of these abilities could be valuable to the right organizations. No doubt you can add more.

Step 3. Cross check your two lists. Which organizations' mission statements and responsibilities seem to fit best with your list of interests, skills, and abilities?

Narrow down your list of organizations to the two or three that fit you the best.

Step 4. Learn more about the organizations on this new short list. If possible, make personal visits. At least call and speak with the volunteer coordinator. What are the organization's precise needs that you might be able to help with, and how many hours a week of your time would be needed?

Step 5. Next, decide just what functions you could perform for each organization and determine how much time you could provide each week on a consistent basis. It might be three times a week for a few hours each day or evening, or once a week for a couple of hours, but the important thing is to choose some substantial contribution that is not too much to handle and is sustainable over time.

Step 6. Finally, after considering the various possibilities, commit yourself to the organization and the volunteer work you feel would best fit what you can offer in skills, effort, and time.

Exercise 2: *Keep a Journal of Your Volunteer Experiences*

Though the idea behind Seva is to serve others selflessly and with no thought of reward, the fact is that the rewards of selfless service are many. As we perform work for others for their sake alone, we find our consciousness expanding and deepening as our appreciation grows for the value of life, other people, and even ourselves.

Assuming that you either already functioned as a volunteer or you enlisted to be one by following the steps in Exercise 1, in this exercise you will keep a journal of your experiences. Each day or evening after your stint as a volunteer, spend at least ten minutes going over your experiences. Put them down on paper. Pay special attention to how your efforts affected the lives of others and how that made you feel. Don't expect that every entry in your journal will necessarily be of a satisfying experience, but it is highly likely that most will. If you find you're too tired on a particular day to write in your journal, you can do it the next day.

The purpose of keeping a journal of your volunteer experiences is to help promote the expansion of consciousness that can come from volunteering. To that end, it is important that you really ponder what memorable things happened that day at your volunteer work. Bring them to consciousness and write them down. Then, to help reinforce whatever lessons you may find yourself learning about Seva, go back and read what you have set down in your journal at the end of each month.

❧

Now

Embrace the Present

"Whereas before you dwelt in time and paid brief visits to the Now, have your dwelling place in the Now and pay brief visits to past and future."

Eckhart Tolle
from *The Power of Now*

It is a mistake to think that Spirit exists far from our day-to-day life. Many spiritual traditions, including Christianity and Hinduism, hold that there is an intimate relation between God or Spirit and everyday life. This relation is clear when we consider the spiritual fulfillment we find when we walk our dharma path. It is even clearer when we think of love and compassion, which is Loving Spirit expressing itself in our relationships. But we can take the lesson even further. Here we will learn how Spirit permeates our lives when we embrace the Principle of Now.

Looked at from one deep perspective, the Now—the present moment—is all that ever exists. The past is a string of Nows that have ceased to be. The future comes into existence as a continuous series of Nows, one after the other. All that ever truly exists is the Eternal Now—the world surrounding us moment by moment. When we plunge into that world with all our heart, when we celebrate and take our stand within it, we infuse our being with the goodness of Spirit. There is no better prescription for spiritual wellness, no more powerful practice for achieving depth, richness, and fullness of life, than to *Embrace the Now.*

Skimming the Surface of the Now

To plunge into the Now is often easier said than done. If you are like most people, you spend an enormous amount of time merely skimming along the surface of the Now. For example, have you noticed how you can drive a car safely along a familiar highway while barely paying attention to the passing scene? Your senses provide information about the pavement and traffic, but you don't really see the trees and houses and businesses you pass by. You barely notice the lovely half moon floating in a vivid blue sky right up there in front of you. Why? Because you're too busy going over all those memories, plans, and concerns that occupy your thoughts.

And this happens not only when you're driving. There are probably many other occasions when you ignore most of what surrounds you Right Here, Right Now because your mind is working overtime. It's called "the monkey mind": your brain engaged in an ongoing silent conversation as if there's a monkey in there (or maybe several) incessantly chattering away.

Thinking, of course, is good and necessary. In fact we have learned, through our consideration of the Principle of Thought, that thinking can be our powerful ally. But like other practices related to wellness, we can carry thinking too far. We pay a heavy price if we allow the remembering and planning and pondering to get out of hand. The more time we spend in our head, the less time we have to enjoy what is before us Right Now. But Now is all we ever have in life. Now is life itself. The very heavy price we pay for too much monkey business is that we find ourselves barely touching the surface of life.

John's Hard Lesson about Participating in the Present

Take John, for example. Wanting to be a good father, he often drives his eager but unathletic daughter Lisa to her soccer games. But until recently, he never really watched her play. Maybe that was partly because Lisa often hesitates to get involved in the real action on the field. Whatever the reason, John typically sat in the bleachers thinking about a million things as his daughter played. He never noticed how she sometimes looked over to see if he was watching her.

One day near the end of the game, Lisa somehow managed to kick the ball past the other team's goal keeper, which resulted in the winning score for her team. As usual, John wasn't paying attention. He was busy trying to decide whether he needed a new lawn mower. After the game, Lisa ran over to ask him if he had seen her make the goal. He lied and said he had. As he looked at his daughter's face beaming with pride, he felt deep sadness. He had missed the only goal she might ever make as a soccer player.

That was when John realized that skimming across the Now was costing him some great experiences and memories with his daughter. At that moment, he made a decision. He still spends a lot of time in his head, but at Lisa's soccer games he puts his monkey mind to rest and embraces the Now.

It is so easy to get carried away in our thinking! Sometimes the mental chatter comes from overly processing the past. Unpleasant memories, regrets, or dreams of the way things used to be replay in our mind over and over, taking us away from the Now. Certainly, we should honor the past and learn from it, but the past exists only as memory traces in our brain, words in books, images in photos. Only Now is ever fully real.

Sometimes it's an imagined future that keeps us in our head and out of the Now. A particularly virulent form of this practice is the rampant urge to "get ahead" that can grip most of a person's thoughts and activities for years or even a lifetime. Yes, we must set goals and make plans. But to achieve them, we must act in the Now. And to allow thoughts of the future to continually obliterate the Now is a terrible mistake. If we constantly dwell on what will be, we are never fully alive to what *IS*. And what is the point of working for Nows that we always ignore when they arrive?

At still other times, concern about what's currently going on in our lives is what keeps us from the Now. *How much is left in the account? What does Greg really think about me? What are we going to do about Denise's report card?* (The voices repeatedly say.) We all have responsibilities to fulfill, people to care for, and goals to achieve. And much of this requires thought. But if we spend all our time thinking about what's on our agenda, there's no time left to embrace the present moment.

Worse, mental chatter is often full of evaluations and judgments about self and others. All day long the mind replays the thought that *nobody here appreciates me.* Or it chews on the idea that *Karen shouldn't wear such a low-cut blouse to work—it's not professional.* Or it thinks dejectedly of how *Sally never says anything nice to me.* Evaluations and judgments are sometimes necessary. For example, we must evaluate our past attitudes and actions in order to learn from them and live more fully in the Now. But evaluations also filter and blur our experience. Instead of the world appearing to our senses in all its vivid complexity, it appears dull and washed out due to our evaluative thoughts. The song of the bird is barely heard. The colors of the sky, the grass, and the flowers are hardly seen. Touches and smells and tastes are barely sensed as the evaluative chatter in our head deadens our appreciation of what is before us at this moment.

Plunging into the Now

The daily miracle of our lives is that we are alive—Right Here, Right Now. To live fully in this miraculous Now, we must plunge into it. We do that by calming the chatter of our minds and opening ourselves fully to what our senses reveal about the world surrounding us at this instant. Opening ourselves in this way is essential, because to embrace the Now, we must be *in* the Now. We have to take the plunge.

So let's do that. For the next few minutes, I would like for you to close your book and closely attend to what you see, hear, feel, smell, and taste right where you are, Right Now.

In preparation, whether you're sitting, lying, or standing, first get comfortable. Then take several slow, deep breaths. Each time, as you exhale, say to yourself, "Just be here now." As you breathe in and out, realize that there is nothing else to do at this moment but just Be Here Now.

Once your mind is calm, listen carefully to whatever sounds are present. Is it very quiet where you are? Or can you detect the murmur of traffic outside, rain on the roof, or voices from the next aisle? What do you hear?

Look at what surrounds you. Allow your eyes to become saturated by the colors and shapes that are present. Notice how varied they are, how brilliant or subdued, how sharp or graceful.

Do you detect any nearby smells—sweet or sour, fresh or stale, perhaps something cooking or an air freshener? And what is the texture of whatever you are touching at the moment: your clothes, your chair, the floor, the pages of the book, its cover?

Is there anyone nearby, a loved one, friend, or stranger? If so, try not to stare, but attend to the expression on his or her face. What do you see there in the lines and surfaces, the shadows and highlights? Happiness? Alertness? Worry?

Is there a pet there with you, maybe a dog or cat or hamster? If so, focus on how sleek or fluffy the animal's coat is, how pink or black or gray the nose. Do you see different shades of color as its coat catches the light?

Using all your senses to take in what surrounds you, continue to let the Now permeate your consciousness for several minutes before you resume reading.

As you did this exercise, I hope you took in the richness and complexity of your surroundings. This wealth and variety are what we miss when we spend too much time in our head. An incredible Table of Reality is always set before us. That's what the monkey mind is skimming over. It's like being at a marvelous feast with countless delicious dishes—but they're covered with the plastic wrap that consists of our thoughts. To plunge into the Now is to rip away the plastic, revealing the splendid Reality that beckons us at every moment.

When you open your senses as you did in the exercise, you receive much more than information. You discover the beauty, variety, and fullness of the world Right Now; you recognize it as *your* world; and you fall in love with the miraculous Reality that presents itself to your senses. What you fall in love with is . . . *a deep blue sky kissing the crowns of the trees in the back yard; the light from the window dancing off the dark shining wood of the table; the sure, safe sound of the heater or air conditioner kicking in; the smell of savory soup simmering on the stove. And then there's the cat's graceful leap onto the window sill, the laugh lines around your mother's mouth as she sits reading, your son's bright eyes as he tells you what happened at recess today. And don't forget your wife's cordial smile as she leans on a door jamb talking with you, or your husband's quiet, satisfied sigh as he sets his briefcase or lunchbox on the table, happy to be home.*

Sensory Meditation

As we learned earlier, meditation is an excellent way to calm the turbulence of the mind. It can also help remove the screen that may be preventing you from fully embracing the world Right Now. What I call *sensory meditation* is especially valuable in helping you plunge into the Now, as I asked you to do just above. For sensory meditation generally the idea is to focus on your bodily experiences and perceptions while you are performing some activity. Don't judge or evaluate or try to understand the meaning of your experiences, just *experience* them as fully as you can. Focus on the shapes and colors your eyes bring to you, the sounds your ears capture, and so on with touches, smells, and tastes.

Don't try to meditate while you are performing any activity, such as driving, for which the meditation could get in the way and make the activity dangerous. But you can often practice sensory meditation while you are doing other things, such as shopping, vacuuming the floor, or gardening. While you are meditating in this way, if other thoughts enter your mind, try not to get wrapped up in them. Let them go and return your attention to what you see, hear, touch, smell, and taste, as well as your bodily feelings. You can learn more about sensory meditation and explore it for yourself in the first exercise at the end of this chapter.

Celebrate the Now

To plunge fully into the Now is to celebrate it. A celebration is an occasion that honors something or someone. It is also an event where everyone has a good time. Think of weddings, birthdays, and New Year's Eve. It is no different when we celebrate the Now, except the celebration is ongoing. What we honor is the Now itself—the wondrous world that our senses bring to us. We honor the fact that we are alive and guests at the superb and amazing party of life. At this party family, friends, and strangers pass through our lives moment by moment—each person infinitely deep, complex, and priceless. To appreciate their singular reality is to honor and celebrate their presence in our world. We also honor our self, for it is *our* world that we celebrate. If we find beauty and mystery and wonder in it, that is partly our doing—it means we are paying attention!

Plunging into the Now is not a passive process. It is one in which we are very engaged with the present moment. We plunge even deeper when we actively step out into the world. By opening ourselves to new places, people, and experiences, we enrich our lives immeasurably. Expanding our world also helps us to appreciate our usual surroundings and view them with new eyes and ears.

I recently traveled up the Pacific Coast Highway to a meeting in San Francisco. I had not traveled that route for some time, and I found the beaches, mountains, and sea to be more beautiful than ever. I stopped more than once to take in the scene Right Here, Right Now. I did not just witness the scene, I was fully within it. I felt myself soaring with the seagulls and rolling in with the waves. At the meeting, I learned that the speaker I had come to hear would not be there. This information barely fazed me because my trip up had been so enjoyable. I could hardly wait to get back on the road to view the route from a new direction. Though a business trip, it was for me a refreshing two-day vacation, an occasion for true celebration.

Facing Death and Living in the Now

As I explained in the preface, there was a time not long ago when I felt close to death due to some serious medical complications. (I am happy to report that all is well now.)

That perceived near-encounter with death had some powerful effects on me, all of them good. One is that it helped strengthen my purpose in life. Another is that it led me to appreciate the present moment more than ever.

I have heard this from others—that a close encounter with death can lead one to savor life's moments more than ever before. I think this happens partly because if we feel we are on death's doorstep, we suddenly realize how much we may soon lose: the colors of the first daffodil or tulip we see in the spring, a cool breeze blowing through our hair on a summer day, the comforting feel of the bed sheets when we are tired, the sound of a child's lilting laughter, and thousands of other everyday experiences.

When we find that we have managed to escape death, we realize we have another opportunity to experience these wonderful moments in the Now, and we luxuriate in that ability. As if we have gained new, super-sensitive eyes, ears, and other sensory organs, we are eager to go out into the world to take in its beautiful colors and sounds, its smells and touches and tastes.

We know that eventually death will come, and we can believe that something good and great lies beyond, but in the meantime we realize what a glorious world we now live in. Hungry again, we want to experience the world Right Here, Right Now to the fullest.

Taking Your Stand in the Now

To take your stand in the Now means putting what has gone before in its proper place. It means to refrain from compulsively mulling over past mistakes, misfortunes experienced, or opportunities missed. It means not wallowing in the past. Our proper job in regard to the past is to learn from it and then use that knowledge to enhance our wellness Right Now.

To take our stand in the Now also means to put the future in its proper place. It means realizing that we must attend to whatever task may be before us Right Here, Right Now if we are to work effectively for future Nows. Visualizing and believing we can achieve our goals can help us do so, but it is our actions in the Now that are most crucial to success. The more we focus on performing the task before us, the more effective will be our efforts. The ideal is to experience the wonderful state of "flow" in which we become so focused on the task that we feel ourselves to be one with it, whether we are building a brick wall, playing a piano, or developing a business proposal. This is another way of plunging into the Now. We lose ourselves there in a process that is pure pleasure.

To take our stand in the Now is to put what has been and what will be in their proper perspectives. All of our past and all of our future intersect in the Eternal Now. Whether we are enjoying the delicious feast set before us at each moment, focusing intensely on the task at hand Right Now, or using knowledge of our past to inform our present, Now is where we must take our stand.

Spirit IS Now

What we find when we plunge into the Now is goodness, beauty, wonder, and truth—the perennial spiritual values that infuse our lives with hope and meaning. However you conceive of Spirit, whether as a Supreme Being, Brahman, Love, Nature, or in some other way, Spirit permeates the Now, filling it with immeasurable goodness. Observe the simple daisy making a place for itself on your lawn, listen to the crickets out past the road at dusk, see how the moon lightens the clouds streaming across its face—in each case, Spirit is using your eyes and ears, Right Here, Right Now, to show itself.

What I hope you take from the discussion of this principle is that Now is all we ever truly have, and how we approach the Now determines the tenor and music of our existence. If we do not learn to embrace the present moment, we will miss out on many beautiful seasons of our lives. It has been said that life passes like a lightning flash. To know that this is true, look at your own past: your childhood or, if you are older, your youth. Where did it go? Wasn't it just yesterday that you were being pushed on a swing, dancing in the high school gym, graduating from college, or walking down the aisle? The years since then went by in a flash, did they not? And so it will be with the next set of decades. This is the time to commit yourself to living your remaining years in your only home, the world Right Here, Right Now.

Set aside an abundance of Nows for your family, friends, the dog, the mountains, the valleys, the smell of roses, the taste of well-brewed tea, and the countless other treasures that pass through your life. In your work, lose yourself in absorbing, joyful Nows. The memories of the times you spend with your family and friends, or out on your own enjoying nature and the world, or focusing on a task in the Now as you strive for worthwhile goals, those memories are what you will be left with at the end of your life. Those memories will tell you who you were and what you valued. If you embrace the Now and make the memories many, and full of love, you will enhance your wellness in all dimensions and nourish yourself splendidly for your older years.

EXERCISES FOR PRINCIPLE 9: NOW

Exercise 1: *Explore Sensory Meditation*

As I explained above, sensory meditation is an excellent way to remove the screen preventing us from fully embracing the world Right Now. It is also a way to calm your mind when you are unable to make a few minutes for sitting meditation. Again, I want to emphasize not to try sensory meditation when you must focus your attention closely on what you are doing for the sake of safety or the quality of your performance. For example, don't try sensory meditation while you are driving a car, walking across a street, or playing tennis. That said, there are plenty of occasions when you can practice sensory meditation. For instance, while you walk your dog along a sidewalk, brush your teeth, or rake leaves, sensory meditation can be appropriate. Let's look at a couple of more examples to explain how you can go about sensory meditation. For the first, consider walking through a park.

As you stroll through the park, you may begin by paying attention to the pressure against your shoes of the surface you are walking on. If you're on a pathway, notice whether the surface feels hard or resilient, smooth or pebbly. If there is grass nearby, is it green or brown, and are there different shades of the predominant color? What do you smell? The scent of evergreens, or of flowers or mint growing beside your path? Are you aware of any sounds, such as traffic outside the park, birdsong, or the buzz of conversation among nearby people? Focus in on these sounds and try to experience them fully. Sit down on a park bench you find along the way. Feel how the pressure of your feet against the pathway suddenly becomes lighter. At the same time, experience how the wood or metal of the bench is pressing against your thighs. Does the bench's surface feel cool or warm, comfortable or uncomfortable? As you fully experience and appreciate what it is like to walk through the park, quietly celebrate the entire complex experience. As you do, your other mental chatter will tend to subside.

If you make this example real by actually practicing sensory meditation as you stroll through a park, you may well find that you experience the park, or at least parts of it, more completely than ever before.

Here's another example—drinking a cup of coffee or tea:

Before you commence drinking, attend to the pressure of the cup against your fingers. Look into the cup and note the colors you see. Smell the brew's aroma. Notice the smoothness of the cup as you bring it to your lips; then feel the liquid rushing into your mouth and past your teeth, bathing your tongue. Pay attention to the taste, whether smooth or bitter, and feel the sensations in your throat as you swallow. Over the next few minutes, fully experience and appreciate what it is like to drink a cup of coffee or tea. Pay attention to as many aspects as you can of the entire process. As you do so, the mental chatter will tend to dissipate and disappear right along with the liquid.

Again, if you make this example real, you may find that you experience your drinking of a cup of coffee or tea more completely than ever before.

As with sitting meditation, while you are practicing sensory meditation, if thoughts enter your mind other than your present sensory experience, don't get wrapped up in them. Let them go and return your attention to your bodily feelings and what you see, hear, touch, smell, and taste at the moment.

Once you have gotten the hang of sensory meditation, your further exercise is to try it two or three times a day for a total of about ten minutes each day. You can practice while eating lunch, raking leaves, sewing, and in many other situations. Do this for one week. For week two, practice for a total of twenty minutes a day, and for week three thirty minutes per day. Not only will this help calm your mind, as you continue to practice you will likely find yourself paying closer attention to the world you experience even when you are not consciously doing sensory meditation.

Exercise 2: *Tame Your Monkey Mind*

As discussed earlier, what gets in the way of living in and appreciating the Now is our monkey mind—all that chatter in our head that goes on constantly as we move through our day. The chatter is made up of judgments, memories, images, feelings, and snatches of self-conversation that flow constantly through our stream of consciousness as we deal with one thing or another. It can be difficult to turn away from these bits of flotsam and jetsam for a few minutes and simply appreciate whatever experience we are having. One reason it can be difficult is that we don't even realize our monkey mind is in control and carrying us along on a rush of thoughts and images. If we learn to identify the monkey mind when it is in operation, we are in a better position to say to it, "Hey, pipe down for awhile while I just enjoy the world in front of me." This second exercise is about learning to catch your monkey mind in the act of being a chatterbox.

The exercise is best done on a day you are not working at your job, whatever it may be. This is because it's true for all of us that to exercise our skills at work, we typically have to be guided by our perceptions and thoughts, and we have little time to just relax mentally and enjoy the world around us. So pick a day when you are relatively free, and pick the entire day because this exercise is intended to go from your waking to your bedtime.

The essence of the exercise is for you to observe the activities of your mind as best you can throughout the day, and as you catch yourself thinking about something, entertaining a memory, silently talking to yourself, or feeling a particular mood or sensation, then write down what you observed. Afterward, go back to whatever you were doing. Do this for an entire day and you will likely be surprised at how often you catch your train of thought traveling quickly down rails you were barely aware of.

If you have to drive somewhere during the day, use a table saw, or perform any other action that needs your undivided attention in order to do safely, then suspend the exercise for that period. And don't do the exercise while watching TV or a movie, or while reading a book, because there's too much informational input going on for you to be trying to observe the workings of your mind at the same time. The exercise works best if you are doing something that allows your mind to wander safely, such as taking a walk, visiting the zoo, shopping, doing simple crafts, or working at household or garden chores such as doing the laundry or watering plants.

Once in awhile as you perform this exercise try to step out of your stream of consciousness for a moment. Experience what exists within your consciousness when the chatter is not providing a silent soundtrack. Can you do it? Sounds easy, but it's difficult for many. Keep trying.

At the end of the day, review your notebook and your experience. Are you surprised at how nimble your mind is, hopping from one subject or feeling to another? Were you able to step away from the chatter for a few minutes and just feel and see and hear the world around you without a film of thought being placed over it?

You may have noticed that in some ways, this exercise is the perfect complement to the first exercise about sensory meditation. The purpose of that exercise was to get you directly into the Now. The purpose of this one is to help get you into the Now by bouncing off of your monkey mind.

ଔ

Gratitude

Shower the World with Gratitude

*"If the only prayer you say in your entire life is
'thank you,' that would suffice."*
Meister Eckhart
quoted in *A Bucket of Surprises* by J. John and M. Stibbe

Spirit displays itself in countless amazing ways for which we can give abundant thanks. From the daffodils that raise their colorful heads to announce the new spring, to the fuzzy caterpillar crossing our path on its way to fulfill its dazzling destiny, to the rising full moon that streams the dark ocean with a path of silver light—we only have to open our eyes to find ourselves surrounded, at every turn, by astonishing goodness and beauty deserving of our deepest gratitude.

The Ability to Feel Gratitude

Even so, there are millions, perhaps even billions of people on our planet who rarely, if ever, take a moment to appreciate and give thanks for the marvelous reality in which they find themselves embedded. This was not always so. When we were children, most of us luxuriated in and appreciated the "ordinary" treasures of each day—the touch of the warm morning sun when we first went outside to play; the taste of our favorite sandwich, just-baked cookies, or a tomato fresh off the vine; the thrilling sight of a thundercloud mushrooming high above us or of an African lion at the zoo. When we were kids, we understood that a new world of bountiful gifts is created for us each day, and we felt its generous reality deep in our bodies and emotions. As a result, we experienced a welcoming sense of appreciation for the world, an appreciation that was our innocent and honest way of saying "Thank you."

As we matured, however, many of us "outgrew" this early sense of glad engagement with reality. A kind of amnesia set in as we lost ourselves in the cares and responsibilities of adulthood. But if we lost ourselves, it was in our minds only, not in actuality. Because whether we feel it now or not, we are still immersed in the raw beauty and sweetness of the world we knew back then. And even if we have lost some of that childhood feeling, we are still the same beings as we were before: privileged children of the Universe and of Spirit.

Next to love, approaching the past and present with gratitude may be the purest way of expressing and feeling our connection to Spirit. To give thanks for what we are given is a pure, gentle, and very powerful way of relating to the world around us. For this reason, the Principle of Gratitude is one of the most profound spiritual ideals for guiding our lives:

> *Shower the world and its many blessings with appreciation and gratitude.*

I am a good example of someone who ignored this fundamental principle for a time. Like most of us, I had a childhood of discovery and wonder. Sometimes I spent the entire day out in the world from daybreak to twilight, enjoying the sun, the rain, the birds, the frogs, and of course my friends. But as I grew and began focusing on my studies, I had less time for other things and started barely appreciating the world around me. Perhaps that was understandable, as I had to work hard to become a physician. What was not so understandable is that once I achieved my goal, I continued for years to focus too hard on "getting ahead," "proving myself," and "making it." And in doing so, I treated the world as merely a backdrop, a foregone conclusion, failing to see it as the miracle it actually is. In my mind at least, I had stepped away from my intimate connection to Spirit and the beauty and goodness of the earth that is my home.

But thankfully, I once again started to understand my connection to the universe surrounding me. And in doing so, I found it even more wondrous than what I knew as a child. Today, if someone were to ask me what is there in the world to appreciate, I would begin by saying that just to have been born into this amazing reality is worth our deepest gratitude. And it is not just the natural world that we are privileged to be part of. The human-made world is also full of wonders that we too often take for granted. Culturally, we are the beneficiaries of great music, books, art, and entertainment. Technologically, we are in an increasingly astounding reality. As I sit at my computer, the world's largest library of information is at my instantaneous command. The cell phone attached to my belt enables me to speak to my wife, children, and friends no matter where they may be. I go into the bathroom to wash my face and remember that in pioneer days, the "plumbing" consisted of a bucket of rainwater and a little house out in the back that must have seemed a long walk on a frigid winter day. Technology has created for us a warm, comfortable world that has made daily living more and more pleasurable. All of these advances warrant our heartfelt thanks.

Gratitude for Others

But what deserves our gratitude most of all is the people in our lives. Too often, we look through people or just see the surface. And this even includes our family and friends. As we become accustomed to them and fall into patterns of behavior, many of us forget to look below the surface and appreciate the complex individual who is there. For instance, many spouses seldom show their appreciation for one another. They neglect to compliment each other, to show their gratitude, to say, simply, "Thank you for being here, for being my wife (or husband), my dearest friend." What a breath of sweet fresh air would be infused into some marriages if the spouses decided to set aside an evening once every two or three months to express their spoken appreciation for one another. They could do this as a part of going out to dinner together, eating a special meal at home, or even just sitting together complimenting, appreciating, and thanking each other for their specific qualities and actions.

And it is not only our family and good friends that deserve our appreciation. According to the Principle of The Virtues of Heart, everyone we meet is infinitely deep, infinitely rich. Even for a co-worker or a casual acquaintance, to voice our appreciation for some aspect of that person's being is a blessing to both the person and ourselves.

The Blessings of Gratitude

The naturalist Joseph Wood Krutch once commented, "Happiness is itself a kind of gratitude," and he was correct, for happiness and gratitude are closely connected. Think of how you feel when someone gives you

The Spiritual Ego Again

In the discussion of the Principle of Seva, we learned that the spiritual ego is present whenever we selflessly work for the benefit of others. The spiritual ego is also present when we feel gratitude for the world and its many blessings.

In both cases, when we practice Seva and when we are quiet and observant, letting wondrous reality reveal itself to our senses, we feel ourselves expanding, becoming more than we were. No longer do we feel locked inside ourselves, separate from others and the world, as if our eyes are windows through which we observe but cannot truly touch what we see. When our spiritual ego expands, the windows disappear, we throw open the door to reality, and we burst into the world to wander joyfully through its many gardens, embracing other souls by showing them kindness and genuine concern for their well-being.

The more we acknowledge Spirit and allow it into our lives, the more our spiritual ego develops. In fact, all of the spiritual principles that we have learned about are meant to help strengthen and expand the spiritual ego. Of those principles, one of the most powerful for self-expansion is to *shower the world and its many blessings with appreciation and gratitude*. To do so is to love the world, and love, as we know, is the very essence of joyful, open, blessed Spirit.

a thoughtful gift or acts in a truly generous way toward you. Isn't the sincere feeling of gratitude that wells up inside a kind of happiness? Or think of a time when you felt joyful, perhaps when you got some good news about your child or a friend. Wasn't that sense of joyfulness you experienced a feeling much like gratitude?

When we are happy, we have a sense of well-being, so it is no surprise that gratitude is a powerful medicine that promotes wellness in all dimensions. For one thing, it puts us firmly on the side of life. When we approach each day with a sense of thankfulness, it is hard for things to get us down. As a result, gratitude has important physiological benefits. It reduces stress, which we know is a potential killer. Fear and worry wash off us like suds in a shower when we plunge into and appreciate what is before us. Studies also show that approaching life with a thankful attitude improves immune system functioning, so vital to good health.

How felicitous that such a gentle and agreeable feeling, the sense of gratitude, can provide powerful physiological benefits! Those who feel no gratitude are too much wrapped up in their own thoughts, desires, and problems. We reach outside ourselves when we approach the world with gratitude, just as we do when we exercise love and the other Virtues of Heart. When we offer a sincere "Thank you" for the good things in our lives, we feel ourselves expanding beyond our narrow ego. When we walk up to a flowering apple tree, smell the blossoms, and touch the new petals, all in appreciation and gratitude for the apple tree's reality, we enlarge our consciousness so that the flowering tree becomes a part of our psyche at that moment. And for as long as we remember it, it will continue to be part of us.

It is true that for people who face very difficult circumstances, it can sometimes be difficult to appreciate and give thanks for the world they are living in. Though they may mouth such words, they do not feel them. But if they could find a way to look past their troubles for a while and see the goodness that still exists in their life, that change in viewpoint could provide them greater strength to deal effectively with their situation.

Gretchen's Gratitude

The power of gratitude to make a positive difference in the life of a person facing great difficulties is well illustrated by the experience of a woman I will call Gretchen.

Gretchen had three children, two girls and a boy, separated by five years. When the oldest girl, Ada, was ten, she developed a form of cancer. Over a period of a year, Ada received a number of difficult chemotherapy treatments at a cancer research hospital, often having to stay several weeks at a time. During that period, Gretchen was full of anxiety and angst at the fact that her daughter was ill and suffering. She was also very angry. She was furious at God, Fate, and the Universe itself, for it seemed to her extremely unjust that such a terrible disease had befallen her daughter.

Though Gretchen tried to exhibit a brave attitude for Ada while visiting at the hospital, her deep-seated anger was difficult to hide, and she was sometimes short with nurses and even doctors, wanting so badly for Ada to get well. When she had to leave her daughter at the hospital and go home, she would lapse into a dark, despairing mood. Her husband Carl tried his best to comfort her, but she was inconsolable. She had little energy for her other two children, Becky and Joshua, so it mostly fell to Carl to entertain them and help with their homework. As for appreciating the rest of the world around her, Gretchen had virtually nothing good to say about it.

What brought Gretchen even further down, at least temporarily, was the fact that on one of her stays at the hospital with Ada, a social worker asked to talk with her. In their meeting, the social worker said she wanted to explore with Gretchen ways to defuse her anger. She said that Gretchen's resentment was working against Ada's recovery because Ada could sometimes feel her mother's emotion and believed that Gretchen was angry at her for having the cancer.

Upon hearing this, Gretchen burst out crying and shouted, "I'm not angry at Ada! It's the damn disease!" She stormed out of the room, emotionally devastated. She realized that though she had been trying to put on a positive face for Ada, it had not been working. She arrived home that evening with only dark thoughts. What bit of good was there in the world, she wondered. What was there to be thankful for? Nothing, nothing, nothing.

The next day was a sunny Saturday, and Gretchen, though still in a desolate mood, forced herself to spend some time with Becky and Joshua out in the yard. The children played quietly, wary of their mother's state of mind. As Gretchen sat on a garden swing watching the children, she noticed that the sunlight filtering through their hair left it almost glowing. As she continued observing the two children, she saw, for the first time in months, how beautiful Becky and Joshua were, playing innocently, obviously trying not to disturb her. Suddenly, her heart was filled with a sense of gratitude that these two dear children were safe, healthy, and strong. It was almost a joyful feeling, though not complete joy, because the ache of what her other daughter was undergoing was still there. But the feeling of gratitude, a sweet warmth, continued to course through her body—gratitude for her two youngest, gratitude for Ada being so strong and fighting her hardest, gratitude for the doctors and nurses who she knew were trying their best.

At that moment, little Becky ran over to Gretchen and said, shyly, "Mommy, I love you." Tears welled in Gretchen's eyes as she realized how much she loved Becky. At that instant, the anger she had felt for so long left her, and all that was left was love and thankfulness for her children, her husband, the medical staff at the hospital, and even herself. "I love you too, Sweetheart," she said, picking Becky up to sit beside her.

Seeing this, Joshua ran to his mother. "Momma," he said. "Will Ada come home soon?"

"I don't know for sure, baby," Gretchen replied as she picked Joshua up so he too could sit beside her. "But I hope so. And I think so. I really do."

The following Monday, Gretchen left again to stay with Ada for several days, leaving Becky and Joshua in the care of their father. As she approached Ada's room, she told herself, "Now you be strong, woman! You be happy for that little girl in there! You give her your love in the form of every bit of strength and positivity you can muster."

A moment later, Gretchen entered the room with a smile brighter than any her daughter had witnessed on her mother for almost a year. And Ada answered her mother with the most luminous smile Gretchen had ever seen in her life.

Gretchen's experience helps us realize that even in dark times, there are always a multitude of things to be thankful for. When we focus on what's wrong, it can be difficult to see what's right. But when we can call to mind what continues to be good in our world, this change in viewpoint can afford us a degree of peace and of strength to endure whatever difficulties we are facing.

Gretchen's story also helps us understand that approaching the world with gratitude is not a matter of being a Pollyanna. At times, each of our lives is visited by trials, troubles, even sometimes tragedy. Because of this, our joys may sometimes be tempered by sadness. Yet these two types of feeing may blend into one deep, bittersweet appreciation of the world that helps us to understand the preciousness of each day, each hour.

As an aid to approaching the world with gratitude, it can help to keep a gratitude journal. Research about gratitude conducted by Professor Robert Emmons at the University of California-Davis showed that people who kept a weekly record of things they were thankful for had better physical health, exercised more regularly, and felt better about their lives. This comes as no surprise because keeping a gratitude journal can engender positive thoughts and help us realize the many things that are going well in our lives.

A way to take this research to heart and practice the Principle of Gratitude would be to dedicate a journal or notebook to making a daily list of five things you are thankful for that occurred on that day or the day before. In fact, this is one of the exercises for you to do at the end of the chapter. If you have trouble listing several things to be thankful for, then you're probably not paying close attention, because we each have countless things to be thankful for every day. As I mentioned, there was a time when I did not realize this clearly, but now I know that even if I were destitute, I would have much to be thankful for: this breath I take, this pulse in my veins, the smell of dust kissed by a first raindrop as I walk along. Do these seem like small things? Are breaths and pulses small things? Where would I be without them? Where would I be without rain?

Another of the exercises below will help you hone your ability to appreciate and give thanks by extending a compliment to at least three people you meet every day. When you do that sincerely, it not only gives the other person a lift, it immediately takes you out of yourself, expands you, and makes you feel lighter and brighter. Be sure to not just mouth the words, say them sincerely. If you can't find something true and complimentary to say about someone, that probably says more about you than about the other person.

Practicing the Principle of Gratitude opens our eyes to the many "small" blessings we enjoy each day and helps us realize that actually, there are no small blessings in this world. Everything is precious. It also helps us to approach the world with enthusiasm. Spirit means for us to exhilarate, relish, and savor the world, to approach our day with fervor and appetite. It is good to take pleasure in what we eat, drink, and do—to enjoy our sleep and our waking each morning to a new day.

As we have learned, too many people, too often, feel as if they are fighting the world. But the world is not our enemy. It is our home. We learned earlier that acceptance of reality is a step toward blessedness. The next step is to go beyond acceptance and approach the world with appreciation and gratitude. By doing so, we immerse ourselves deeper into the beauties and wonders of the River of Life.

We have also learned that we create much of our reality by our thoughts and how we approach the world. When we appreciate the world as it is and give thanks for what we are given, we are in fact walking hand-in-hand with Spirit, to help create a blessed world—a world full of light and love, a world of beauty, compassion, courage, love, and openness all around us.

EXERCISES FOR PRINCIPLE 10: GRATITUDE

Exercise 1: *Keep a Gratitude Journal*

For this exercise, I would like you to keep a daily gratitude journal for one week. The physical journal can be a notebook, reminder, or computer file. Each day, list five things that happened that day or the day before that you are thankful for. Choose a regular time to make your list, perhaps before you leave for work in the morning, at lunchtime, or in the evening before bed. Don't hurry. Give yourself enough time to ponder carefully what has happened yesterday or today for which you are thankful. You may soon find that listing five things is not enough. Choose what you think is a good number for you. You may also find yourself reflecting on things to be thankful for that never or seldom occurred to you before.

I know that when I came to ponder what I was thankful for, I came up with some great things that I had been taking for granted. For example, I realize how thankful I am that on a warm day my car has a very effective air conditioner. I feel gratitude that the waste management workers are always so punctual in picking up the trash. And I am thankful that I no longer have to wait for a week or more to receive a communication from friends or family on the other side of the world. With e-mail, I receive their message almost instantly. There are so many things—important things—to be thankful for each day, it seems that gratitude should be our constant companion.

After performing this exercise for one week, decide whether the practice increases your appreciation of the gifts you are receiving from the World Right Now. It would be marvelous if you were to continue the assignment into the future, at least by setting aside a few minutes of each day to contemplate what you are thankful for that day.

Exercise 2: *Acknowledge Others with Compliments*

Many people, even when they are around others, actually spend much of their time in private, locked in their perceptions and thoughts, trying to balance themselves as they encounter the various challenges the day brings. Their chattering mind is constantly going with thoughts not only about their daily projects, but about various other concerns. Maybe they are trying to figure out what to do about their child's poor grades, attempting to understand the intent of a comment the boss made to them, worrying about the results of a medical test, or anticipating how good it will be to get home because they feel so tired after a poor night's sleep. The matters, both small and large, that can concern us are countless.

Given this, for someone to suddenly break into these private thoughts and offer a sincere compliment can be heartening and refreshing. To give a compliment is to reach out to another person, to acknowledge that you recognize not only that the other person exists, but their worth and goodness. It is a way of saying, "I appreciate the fact that you are you."

And that's what this exercise is about. Your assignment is to extend a sincere compliment to at least three people each day for a week. The compliment can be something as simple as, "You look good with that hair style, Bonnie," or "I like that shirt you're wearing, Tom." It can be a compliment and a sign of gratitude for some longstanding quality or activity, such as "I really appreciate the fact that you are always so easy to talk to," or "I just wanted to tell you that you are a gem for always picking the kids up from practice." If you can offer more than three compliments a day, all the better. The idea of doing this every day for a week is that you will get in the habit of showing your appreciation to others. And it's a great habit to get into.

Can't think of complimentary things to say to people? Try this: the day before you start this exercise, take some time to think about the people who are often in your life and those you meet only occasionally (the bank teller, the dry cleaner), then challenge yourself to formulate and write down some sincere compliments you might pay each one next time you meet them. Then go to it!

PRINCIPLE 11

Cʒ

The Divine You

Recognize Spirit in All of Us

"The world is not divine sport, it is divine destiny. There is divine meaning in the life of the world, of man, of human persons, of you and of me."

Martin Buber
from *I and Thou*

We are living in a time when many people pay, at best, only meager attention to Spirit. When they have occasion to think of Spirit, it strikes them as something other-worldly, far removed from their daily experience. But in actuality, Spirit is as close to us as our eyes, ears, hands, and heart. We see the face of Spirit when we observe the morning glory open its petals to a new day. We hear the voice of Spirit when we listen to the rain falling against the window. We touch Spirit when a cool breeze brushes our cheeks on a hot summer day. And we feel Spirit in our heart when someone greets us with a welcoming smile or we stop to help an elderly person manage a heavy bag of groceries. In those and countless other ways, we are intimately connected to Spirit at every moment of our lives.

More even than that, each of us embodies Spirit, and thereby embodies the Divine.

This will come as news to some, especially if they have put too much store in an old argument whose conclusion is that we humans are insignificant creatures barely worth a nod in "the grand scheme of things." You may have heard the argument, which goes like this: Each of us is only one among billions of creatures who live on a smallish planet orbiting a medium-sized star somewhere in the outskirts of an unremarkable galaxy that contains a hundred billion stars and is only one of a couple of hundred billion galaxies. Therefore, in comparison to the vast panorama that is the universe, we are only "insignificant motes of dust."

By concluding that humans are "insignificant," those who wield this argument apparently mean something more than the obvious fact that we are physically small compared to the universe. But if so, their reasoning is an excellent example of what in logic is called a *non sequitur,* meaning that their conclusion does not follow from their premises. For why should we suppose that our physical size in relation to universe has anything to do with our significance? Is a 100-ton boulder more significant than a five-gram hummingbird? If you want to crush a car it is. But not if you want to observe scintillating beauty on the wing.

But even if we reject this bad argument, we still have to make a case for the idea that we embody Spirit. I want to explain how, for just about any conception of Spirit we may have, it turns out that Spirit exists in each of us. To help make that case, let's look at four of humankind's main spiritual conceptions.

Four Ways of Viewing Spirit

One of the world's chief conceptions of Spirit is the idea of a personal God. That there is such a God is the view of the Christian, Jewish, and Sunni Muslim faiths, among others. Though there are many differences among these religions, they have in common the belief in a God who created the physical universe but also transcends the universe by being totally independent of it. However, most adherents of these religions also believe that God is present in the physical world. And many believe that God somehow exists within each person who believes in him. For example, in Christianity, the biblical verse of 1 Corinthians 6:17 says, "But whoever is joined to the Lord becomes one spirit with him." This and other biblical passages, including ones that speak of a person's body being a temple of the Holy Spirit, indicate that in some way, God exists in those who believe in God. On this conception, we are not beings whose reality is exhausted by the fact that we have material bodies. We are beings who are able to embody Spirit, understood as a personal God.

We can illustrate this idea with the words of Elaine, a young Christian woman who explains her personal interpretation of God's presence by saying she believes that when she silently prays to God, she is not praying to a divine being who exists in some other place or dimension, but rather to a divinity who is actually present within her.

"God is everywhere," she says, "which means God is here with me, too. But it's even more than being with me. I feel that God is actually in me, in my heart and soul, everywhere I go, at every moment."

For those who feel the same way, Spirit, understood as a transcendent God, is also a personal God who is immanent within them.

A similar conclusion can be drawn in the case of another conception of Spirit, one that is common in Hinduism. This is the idea that Spirit is identical to Brahman, which is held to be the highest reality. The concept of Brahman is more abstract than that of the Christian or Jewish God. At least for many who practice Hinduism, Brahman is not viewed as a personal deity, or even as an individual being. Brahman is understood to be the transcendent source and ground of all things, the fundamental spiritual reality. Yet Spirit as Brahman is also thought to be immanent in our lives, for Hindus hold that Brahman touches each of us intimately. This is because the nature of fundamental spiritual reality is consciousness, which is also our own nature. In fact, we are conscious only because we partake of the fundamental consciousness that is Brahman.

Sunil, a middle-aged Hindu man, explains this conception further by saying that if we were able to understand who we truly are, we would discover that the private ego that we each seem to have is actually an illusion. Our true nature is that we are united with Brahman. He uses the metaphor of Brahman being like an ocean.

"This ocean is fundamental consciousness," he says, "and it is the sum total of everything. There is nothing that is not Brahman. If we could understand our own true nature, we would realize that each one of us is like a wave or a ripple on that ocean. That is how closely connected we are to Brahman."

Given this understanding, it is evident that it is an understatement to say that in Hinduism we have an intimate relation to Brahman. It is closer to say that on this conception, we are identical with Spirit.

A third basic view of Spirit is to identify it with nature or physical reality. The great physicist Albert Einstein exemplified this view. Though Einstein rejected traditional religion, his writings make clear that he often thought of the physical universe as a kind of mystical, yet rational reality. His words show that he regarded the natural world with a degree of awe that is reminiscent of the way many people think of whatever God they may believe in:

"Try and penetrate with our limited means the secrets of nature and you will find that, behind all the discernible concatenations, there remains something subtle, intangible and inexplicable. Veneration for this force beyond anything that we can comprehend is my religion. To that extent I am, in point of fact, religious" (quoted by H. G. Kessler in *The Diary of a Cosmopolitan*).

Einstein also regarded the uncovering of nature's mysteries as a sacred occupation. He put it this way: *"My religion consists of a humble admiration of the illimitable superior spirit who reveals himself in the slight details we are able to perceive with our frail and feeble mind"* (quoted by P.A. Bucky and A. Weakland in *The Private Albert Einstein*). For these reasons, it is clear that Einstein—and others who think similarly—felt and feel a spiritual connection to the physical universe.

But is Einstein's idea of Spirit one in which humans actually embody Spirit? Yes, for two reasons. First, we are intimately related to nature physically because we are parts of nature. And since for Einstein nature embodies Spirit, then on his view we are parts of Spirit. Second, we can have a mental connection to Spirit by uncovering and contemplating its laws and principles. But by doing so, we take them into our own mind, our own self. In that sense, we embody the principles and laws of Spirit understood as nature.

Still another conception of Spirit—perhaps the most abstract of all—is the idea that perennial values such as Truth, Justice, and Beauty exist as eternal ideals to guide our lives. The Greek philosopher Plato put forth this view over two thousand years ago, and for many people the idea remains fresh and relevant. In fact, the majority of us embrace this view to some degree. For example, most of us believe that there is such a thing as Truth, and we think that living in the truth is something worth doing. We want truth from our leaders, our friends, and ourselves. But if we believe that a value such as Truth is eternal and is also meant to guide our actions, then this amounts to viewing it as both transcendent and immanent in our lives. This double nature makes it, like the other conceptions, a spiritual one. The difference is that here, eternal values play the role of Spirit.

Do those who conceive of Spirit in this way embody Spirit as they understand it? Before addressing this question, we should first recognize that some people combine a belief in eternal values with some other conception of Spirit. For example, people who believe in a personal God can also believe that there are eternal values such as Truth and that these values should guide their lives. But how about people whose only spiritual conception consists of faith in one or more eternal values? On this very abstract conception of Spirit, do people embody Spirit? The answer is clearly yes, if they are actually guided by the eternal values in which they believe, because to be guided by those values is to *embody them* in their actions.

The words of Kelly, a young woman who admits to being non-religious but who is also concerned about raising her two children to exhibit certain values, may help us to better understand this view. In talking about what she wants to teach her children, she says:

"One extremely important thing I want my kids to understand is that acting as a good person should not be contingent on receiving some extraneous reward. Being moral and ethical are rewards in themselves. That may sound old fashioned, but that's what I think. Some of the main values I believe in are that we should respect everyone and be compassionate toward those who are less fortunate. And we should have personal integrity and have the courage to stand up for what we believe. Those are things we should never compromise on. I want my children to honor those values. And the way to honor them is not just to think about them or to mouth them. The only way to honor them is to live them as best they can. In everything they do."

It is evident that Kelly believes strongly in certain enduring values that serve the role of spiritual guideposts. It is also clear that she wants her children not just to believe in those values, but to embody them in their actions throughout their lives.

The Spirit within Us

There are of course other religious and philosophical views about the nature of Spirit, but the four I have briefly spoken about are some of the most common and widespread. They illustrate the great range of spiritual conceptions, from the very personal to the very abstract, that humans have developed over time. For thousands of years, belief in Spirit has been an important aspect of the lives of people throughout the world, with every culture having its own predominant ideas about its nature. And still today, almost every one of us, in his or her way, looks to

Divinity Begins at Home

Sometimes it occurs that a person who has failed to detect the holiness of others will suddenly see it displayed in one particular person. This seems to occur for some people on first meeting the Dalai Lama or hearing him talk. I believe that when this happens, the individual is actually seeing a reflection of his or her own goodness in the Dalai Lama, for we cannot see the holiness in another unless we have that holiness within ourselves. And we all do.

Even if a person has never or seldom before seen the holiness in another, if he or she suddenly sees it in one person, then a beginning has been made. In the future, the individual will be more likely to see it in others: in a child's smile, a father's weathered face, the lines of love around a mother's mouth.

However, the most important place to see holiness is in our own selves. Before we do that, it may be difficult or even impossible to see it in others. But once we do, we cannot help but see that holiness— the tender kiss of Spirit—exists in everyone we meet.

something higher—some transcendent being, reality, or set of values—to help us define and make sense of our lives. In this way we are spiritual beings through and through, which is why a life without any semblance of Spirit is a life that goes against our humanity. What helps further to demonstrate the importance of Spirit in our lives is the fact that for many conceptions of Spirit, including the four we learned about, Spirit is something that we actually embody, something that is inside us.

Throughout this book, I have purposely been noncommittal about the nature of Spirit. I am not here to claim that Spirit takes the form of a personal God, Brahman, nature itself, eternal values, some combination of these, or something else. This is a matter we must each decide for ourselves. However, I have said a few basic things that I believe are true about Spirit.

First, Spirit exists, is eternal, and is good.

Second, Spirit is the essence of wellness, which is of course the main theme and reason for this book.

Third, the essence of Spirit is love, which is why Spirit and Heart are so intimately intertwined and why practicing the Virtues of Heart is so important for wellness in all four of our dimensions.

In this chapter, I have been making a case for the fourth main thing I want to say about Spirit:

> *Spirit abides within each of us and is there to inform our lives if we allow it to do so.*

This means that we each have divinity inside us, every one of us, no matter what our background, circumstances, or even character.

Due to their attitudes and behavior, it may be difficult to accept the idea that Spirit lives within some of the people we come across. But in some, Spirit is still only a seed, longing to be watered and cultivated. At the other pole, there are those for whom Spirit has taken root so completely that it has blossomed wonderfully within them. Occasionally, we may be fortunate enough to come across such a one, and when we do we realize that we are in the presence of love and goodness made flesh. I think of Jesus and the Buddha, and of some in more recent times, such as Mahatma Ghandi, Mother Teresa, and the Dalai Lama.

The great majority of us fall somewhere between these two extremes. Spirit, in most of us, is much more than a mere seed. It is already flowering in our thoughts and actions more than we may realize, though our greatest blossoming is yet to come. This means that we too are love and goodness made flesh.

If it is difficult for you to view yourself as embodying Spirit, then I urge you to seek deeper inside yourself. One great advantage of understanding that we embody Spirit is that it increases our self-acceptance and self-regard, which are among the most important qualities we can possess for living a happy, loving, fulfilling life. A few pages back I objected to a faulty argument whose conclusion is that humans are "insignificant." This is a conclusion that far too many people come to about themselves simply based on various life experiences. For one reason or another, they start believing that their lives are inconsequential and that they themselves are irrelevant. Such a conclusion is totally false and creates great harm. We know that thought can be our powerful ally if we turn away from negative and harmful conceptions of the world and ourselves. We must come to understand that Spirit dwells within us. Because of this, its principles are our own. They serve as a beacon to light our way through the world, empowering us to live in abundant wellness.

Realizing that we are each blessed by Spirit also enables us to recognize the blessedness of others. Those who think they are insignificant typically believe the same thing of other people, and they treat them accordingly. Those who understand that we are all blessed by Spirit are immediately inspired to treat others with respect and compassion. This stands to reason since the essence of Spirit is love. Compassion and kindness toward others cannot help but thrive when we recognize them as embodying Spirit. It is true that the actions of some people seem to indicate that they are not connected to Spirit in any way. But we must try to see through that ruse and recognize the kernel of goodness inside. The sooner we are all able to see the blessedness in one another, the sooner we will all blossom.

If you still have any doubt that you are the locus of Spirit, I hope you will follow the advice of Marcus Aurelius, from *Meditations*:

> *Look within. Within is the fountain of good, and it will*
> *ever bubble up, if thou wilt ever dig.*

Here, the great philosopher and Roman emperor is advising us to reflect on our inner nature. When we calm our mind and reflect deeply about who we are, we will come to understand that it is our nature to be good. And through that very act of digging, goodness, love, and wellness will rise in us like a fountain.

This is the revelation of Spirit. This is Spirit at work.

EXERCISES FOR PRINCIPLE 11: THE DIVINE YOU

Exercise 1: *Investigate Your Connection to Spirit*

For this exercise, find a portion of time, at least a half hour, to think back over your life to the times you have felt the presence of Spirit in some way and, as you do, make a list of these times. There may have been occasions in a church, synagogue, or mosque when you felt that Spirit was with you. There may have been times out in Nature when you felt the presence of Spirit, perhaps while you watched the stars at night or upon waking to a just-risen sun and the songs of birds. Or times when you felt Spirit while you were with someone you love—your child, spouse, or friend. Or perhaps there were other occasions when you felt Spirit somehow present.

There may be a few who say they have never felt the presence of Spirit in anything they have experienced, but I believe that everybody has felt Spirit in their lives at various times even if they didn't recognize it as such. So think hard and try to make a complete list.

Once you've completed your list, examine it to find if there are any commonalities among the incidents or times you have listed. Are most of the occasions somehow related to religion? Do they occur in places of beautiful architecture? Perhaps there is a group of items related to nature, or even some part of nature, such as mountains, skies, stars, animals, or sunrises. Or there may be incidents that are related to family. Do you find that most of the times when you have some experience of Spirit, you are with others, or are you alone?

Also try to describe to yourself what it is like when you feel the presence of Spirit in your life. Is it totally ineffable? Or can you find some words that at least partly describe how you feel at the time? If so, write them down. Ask yourself whether your experience is one of Spirit being somewhere "out there," or somehow inside you. Or is it both? And what happens after these experiences? Do they tend to make you happier or kinder to others? Do they affect your attitudes or behavior in some other way?

The purpose of this exercise is for you to become more aware of how your sense of Spirit tends to occur in your life—when, where, how, and its effects. By better understanding these details, you may feel yourself connecting more closely with Spirit and be more on the lookout for how Spirit touches your life in the future.

Exercise 2: *Contemplate Different Ways You May Embody Spirit*

We have learned four ways people conceive of Spirit (and no doubt there are more): (1) a Supreme Being; (2) Brahman, the fundamental reality; (3) Nature or physical reality, and (4) eternal verities such as Truth, Justice, Courage, and Kindness. For each of these I described how Spirit could be viewed as being embodied in the individual person.

This exercise is about these four conceptions of Spirit. It is not a particularly easy exercise, as it requires you to do some hard thinking. But it is informative, can be expansive, and is potentially even liberating. You will need some quiet time, at least a half hour to an hour. Your job is to entertain each of the four conceptions of Spirit I listed above, one by one; to try to understand, as best you can, the nature of that conception; and then to try to understand how, according to that conception, Spirit can be seen as embodied in people.

Now you may personally favor one of the four conceptions above the others, but I would like you to entertain all of them. So don't assume you know the results of this exercise before doing it. And don't automatically assume that your conception of Spirit must be the only correct one and that all others are totally wrong.

As you do the exercise, you may find yourself concluding that there is at least some truth in each of the four conceptions of Spirit and that there is a sense in which Spirit is embodied in you and other people in more than one way. Maybe even in all four ways. That is for you to contemplate.

PRINCIPLE 12

Cß

Non-Attachment

Live a Spiritual Life

"We are not human beings having a spiritual experience;
we are spiritual beings having a human experience."
Pierre Tielhard de Chardin
from *The Phenomenon of Man*

We have been learning that total wellness in Mind, Body, and Heart requires us to also be well in our spiritual dimension, and that many ills in people's social, psychological, and even physical aspects are due to their not making an honored place for Spirit in their lives. We have also learned a number of principles for promoting wellness in Spirit. But these principles will be of little value if we do not put them into practice. It is not enough to practice them only occasionally and to otherwise neglect them. We must find within ourselves the desire and the will to allow Spirit to inform our lives every day. We must, in short, live a spiritual life.

Does "leading a spiritual life" mean we have to give away our possessions, don sackcloth, and go live in a cave to seek enlightenment? The answer to that question is a resounding *No*. Living a spiritual life is fully compatible with enjoying "worldly" pleasures such as dining, entertainment, sports, and travel. And why shouldn't it be? The world we live in is suffused with Spirit and is here to be appreciated and enjoyed. Leading a spiritual life is not about austerity for the sake of austerity. It is much more a matter of how we think about ourselves and the world we are privileged to live in, how we treat others, and how we deal with our past, present, and future. My purpose here is to focus on how we can fit the spiritual principles we have learned into our day-to-day lives and how, by doing so, we make our "ordinary" lives extraordinary.

Success and Non-Attachment

I spoke earlier of runaway materialism and the unbridled desire to gain more and more possessions, a desire that controls millions of people's lives. As we learned, the problem is not, in itself, money or owning things. The trouble arises when financial and material success becomes a person's supreme value and all other values become secondary. It is only a short step from this idea to thinking that it is all right to violate any other value if it means making more money. When someone believes that values such as honesty, friendship, fidelity, love, kindness, and courage can be thrown under the wheels of the runaway train of materialism, there can be only one final result: a disastrous train wreck that will leave the person ill in all aspects of life. As this is being written, a top news story illustrates just how devastating the train wreck can be. In this case, an individual who deceived trusting friends and other investors for the purpose of bilking them of billions of dollars was found out, had his empire taken away, and was sentenced to a life in prison. His actions also reportedly contributed to the suicides of several people, including one of his own sons. That is a train wreck of epic proportions.

Of course, it is true that some individuals are able to take advantage of others and advance financially without ever being brought to any legal justice. But that certainly does not mean they are getting away "scot free," for it is difficult to imagine they can be happy or even healthy in any true sense. Focused as they are on their own egocentric concerns, sacrificing others' well-being to their greed, their dimension of Heart becomes horribly withered. By isolating themselves from genuine caring human interaction, they create their own stark, inhuman prison.

What such a person fails to realize is that financial success does not require us to subordinate other values to making money. In fact, it is just the opposite. Being guided by spiritual values and principles can actually empower us to create for ourselves and our families a life of material comfort. For one thing, if we follow our dharma path by seeking a career that taps into our natural talents and interests, we greatly increase our chance of material success. This is because when we follow our passion we enjoy what we do and tend to do it very well, which is a major part of the recipe for success.

But won't having a degree of material success put us in danger of falling into the trap of runaway materialism? Not if we understand and follow the Principle of Non-Attachment.

The idea of nonattachment stems from Eastern philosophies that recognized how people's desires to be materially successful can be a source of anxiety, dissatisfaction, and even misery. That's what happens if they begin craving material goals so much that they allow their happiness to depend on their achieving the goals. When we crave something, whatever it may be—a new dress, a new car, a vacation trip—we become attached to it in our mind. Then, if we don't get what we crave or don't get it soon enough, this attachment preys on our thoughts and emotions. We find ourselves continually dissatisfied with the status quo, unable to appreciate whatever blessings we have at the moment as we constantly focus on what we do not have. Even if we are successful in obtaining what we crave, our satisfaction may be short lived if something else whets our appetite. Then we begin craving the new thing and find ourselves unhappy again until we are able to obtain it.

The problem is allowing our mind to become attached to whatever it is that we want to have or to happen. The solution is to follow the Principle of Non-Attachment, which says:

> *Intend what you want, but do not attach to it in your mind.*
> *Do not allow what you do not have to interfere with*
> *enjoying the blessings you do have.*

Following just this one principle can help keep us grounded in the Now as we balance our present reality with our future goals. It can prevent us from craving and grasping for what we do not have to the point that we lose sight of what we do have. Ironically, following this principle can also actually help us obtain whatever it is we intend. This is because realizing that it is no tragedy if we do not get whatever it is we want—that new dress, new car, or vacation—relaxes our mind, enabling us to be more creative in finding ways to fulfill our intention.

For some it can be difficult to follow the Principle of Non-Attachment given the emphasis on material achievement and consumerism that we find in our society. Our entire economic system depends on creating desires for goods and services, and every day new products are introduced to whet

Non-Attachment and Following Your Dharma Road

To some it seems contradictory to learn your purpose in life, to make detailed plans to achieve that purpose, to start down the road toward fulfilling the purpose, but to practice non-attachment while doing so. How is that possible, they ask. The more you desire to achieve the goal, the more you will do to make it a reality, so doesn't not attaching to the goal mean that you do not desire it very much and therefore will not work hard for it?

It is true that non-attachment works against desire, but only against what we can call "grasping desire." Those with grasping desire tend to think that they *must* have the object of desire. If an individual with grasping desire does not obtain the object desired, he or she tends to be unsettled and unhappy.

Non-grasping desire is different. Let me illustrate with my own case. I believe that my proper purpose in life is to be a holistic healer. I want to be that healer. In fact, by offering you this book, I am partly fulfilling that purpose and so I am fulfilling my desire. But I am not grasping after achieving my purpose. If something should happen that would make it impossible for me to achieve that purpose, I would not be devastated. I would simply rethink what my purpose in life should be, and I would begin working toward that.

Often, I evaluate my attitudes toward what I believe is my purpose. If I find that I am worrying too much about the results of my efforts, I remind myself to ease up a bit on my desire. I should always do what I think is best for fulfilling my purpose, but I should always remember that following my purpose is only one aspect of my existence. It is an important one, of course. But it is equally if not more important that I am a husband, a father, a son, a brother, a friend; no matter what happens, I will always be blessed by having these roles. Remembering this helps keep everything in perspective. It helps me work toward achieving my goals, while not attaching to them in a grasping way.

our appetite. Within this context, it can be easy to fall into the trap of constantly wanting the newest, biggest, or best gadget available. It can be hard to not get mentally attached to what we don't have. But it is not inevitable that we do so, and there are many who manage to practice the Principle of Non-Attachment even if they never heard of it before.

Probably the best overall strategy for practicing non-attachment and not falling into the materialism trap is to understand ourselves.

What Do You Stand for?

In the discussion of the Principle of Harmony, we learned the importance of self-knowledge for creating harmony in our lives. Self-knowledge is essential today when we are constantly beset by cross-currents of communication that try to convince us of what we should want, what we should believe, and who we should be. We can become literally lost in those cross-currents as we are buffeted this way and that by a thousand different voices and messages. The best way to find solid ground within these streams of conflicting information is to look inward and take stock of who we are, where we want to go in our lives, and what values we want to uphold. If we do not do so, we are in danger of losing our autonomy and allowing those critical issues to be determined by forces outside us.

Helping you to perform this value inventory has been one main purpose of this book. From the beginning, I have been giving you reasons to believe that nurturing your spiritual aspect is a necessary key to wellness not only in Spirit, but in Body, Mind, and Heart. I have been explaining why wellness, happiness, harmony, and true wealth are not a matter of obtaining more money, possessions, or prestige. Rather, they depend crucially on issues such as how we think about the world; whether we are being true to ourselves; whether we accept and appreciate the beautiful, complex, reality that confronts us each day; and how well we respect and care for others.

Throughout, I have wanted the ideas and principles in this book to serve as tools that you could use to better understand yourself and how you want to conduct your life. They are also instruments to help you realize that when you are guided by spiritual principles, life burns more brightly, with more accomplishment and joy. I thus hope you will set aside the time to take a thoughtful inventory of yourself, where you are in life right now, and what values you want to uphold. As you do so, think about each spiritual idea and principle you have encountered here and how it can fit into and inform your life.

When you do that, one question I would expect you to ask yourself is this: "How do I put together the different lessons I have learned here in order to lead a spiritual life?" I will attempt to answer that question by revisiting and connecting the most important ideas we have talked about.

The Primacy of Mind

One way of contemplating and ordering the lessons in this book is to think of them in terms of two main ideas. The first of these is the idea that Mind, what we think of ourselves and the world, is crucial to our wellness in all dimensions and to our happiness. In the case of self-perception, there is a radical difference between people who believe in themselves and those who do not, as we learned from the story of Tamara and Cindy. The difference shows itself in all dimensions of a person's life. Because of the primacy of our thoughts and attitudes, much of this book has been spent on setting forth a way of perceiving yourself that is empowering, heartening, and true.

This way of viewing yourself has three key aspects. First, you are wonderfully unique. You have a singular personality, with a combination of talents, interests, knowledge, and experience that make you different from all other humans. Second, you embody enormous potential for fulfilling one or more long-term purposes that fit you perfectly—your dharma road. Third, you are, like all of us, a child of Spirit. It is not for me to define Spirit beyond saying that Spirit is great and good, its essence is love, and it is immanent in the world. Other than that, it is up to you to conceive of Spirit in a way that has meaning for you. But however you understand it, you have an intimate connection to Spirit. And because of that connection, you are blessed.

If you took only these three ideas from this book, it would have served a powerful purpose.

But there is much more. How we think of the world in which we are embedded is also a key to our happiness, our achievement, and our wellness. In several places I explained how supposing that reality is somehow against us can be a self-fulfilling prophecy, which is tragic because the world is not against us in any way. Yes, there are dangers in the world, and we therefore must be prudent and wise in our actions. But the world is also full of gifts that provide us with many healthful and enjoyable benefits. It is because nature is a doubled-edged sword that we must learn to work in harmony with the world, as ancient Ayurvedic medicine teaches us.

Those who feel that reality is against them are allowing negative emotions to govern their relationship to the world. Instead of emotionally resisting or fighting reality, the Principle of Acceptance teaches us to accept what is. The River of Life will take us where it will, and to waste our energies trying to swim against it is pointless and destructive of our well-being. Our intention should be to swim *with* the current and use its great power to help take us where we want to go and to create within the world what we want to create.

Acceptance, of course, is only the first step. The world is infused with Spirit every moment of our lives, and to appreciate and celebrate what we are given is a profoundly spiritual practice that promotes wellness in Body, Mind, and Heart. Appreciating and celebrating the Now is an activity that eludes us when we are wrapped up in our evaluations of ourselves, our circumstances, and other people. This mental chatter, the product of the monkey mind, forms the background of much of our experience. We must quiet the monkey at least some of the time and simply attend to the exquisite beauty that permeates our experience. In a word, we must take a joyful *plunge* into the Now, savoring and celebrating the wonders that surround us.

This kind of appreciation breeds gratitude, which is one of the most spiritual of activities. To appreciate the many gifts we are given each day is actually, in itself, a kind of gratitude. The world we experience flows naturally from Spirit, and when we appreciate the song of a bird, a cooling rain, or the welcome face of a friend, we are saying "thank you" to those expressions of Spirit.

The Primacy of Heart

The second main idea that can help put order in the others is the principle that the Virtues of Heart are fundamental to wellness and to living a spiritual life. Love, as we know, is the essence of Spirit. In fact, the truest mark of the presence of Spirit in our lives is the presence of love. You may have experienced the truth of this yourself at times when you looked with unconditional love upon your child, spouse, relative, or friend. At those moments, you experienced deep meaning, which is one of the signposts of Spirit.

Because Spirit is the wellspring of love, to live a spiritual life is, perhaps more than anything, to live a life full of love and friendship, compassion and kindness. It is a life in which we recognize that every person in the world, no matter what their background or situation, is holy, and in which we take to heart Christ's words, ". . . Truly I tell you, whatever you did for one of the least of these brothers and sisters of mine, you did for me" (Matthew 25:40).

While Spirit is love, the opposite of Spirit, as we know, is the selfish ego, whose only concern is fulfilling its own self-centered desires and needs. The selfish ego is, in itself, heartless. Other people are there not to be cared for or appreciated, but to be used. Spirit, in contrast, leads us out of ourselves. Our selfish ego transforms into a spiritual ego as we feel ourselves transcending our narrow self-centered concerns to encompass the reality of others. This promotes wellness in all dimensions of our being. It brings joy and deep meaning to our lives. And it creates a wealth of rich experiences that those who focus only on fulfilling their selfish desires cannot understand. They may think they are living a life full of exciting experiences that the rest of us are missing out on, but they are like one-trick ponies. Their lives are full of constant chasing after experiences that may be gaudy, but are joyless, self-serving, and basically empty. Their lack of genuine caring for other people leaves them fundamentally alone, trapped in the narrow confines of their selfish ego.

Practicing the Virtues of Heart also helps us to adopt other spiritual ideas and principles, including those we discussed in the last section. For instance:

- Because the world lights up and becomes more beautiful when we approach it with love and compassion, any thought that it may be against us is impossible.
- We find it easier to go with the flow of the River of Life and to practice acceptance because we realize that the flow is generous and ultimately benevolent.

- As we expand outward to others, our mind becomes calm so that we can better experience and appreciate whatever beauties and wonders we may encounter in the Now.

- Our self-belief soars when we feel ourselves caring for others because we know we are being empowered by and expressing Spirit.

In these and other ways, practicing the Virtues of Heart can help us to live by the spiritual ideas and principles we have learned about.

And so we have arrived full circle to find that the primacy of Mind and the primacy of Heart are mutually supporting. In fact, all of the spiritual ideas and principles we have learned are interconnected. I hope that as you take stock of where you are right now and where you want to be, you will search for those connections. I leave you with the same thoughts that we began with: To achieve maximum wellness in all dimensions of our lives is a worthwhile and wonderful goal. And there is no better way to move strongly toward that goal than to embrace the principles of Spirit, which is the very essence of wellness.

EXERCISES FOR PRINCIPLE 12: NON-ATTACHMENT

Exercise 1: *Learn More about Your Strengths and Values*

Living a spiritual life is living a life infused with values. Whether those values are consciously entertained, or so engrained that they are barely conscious, they guide our actions. In Exercise 2 at the end of the chapter on the Principle of Harmony, you addressed the question of which values you consider most important. Here, you will continue along that line, learning more about what values guide your life. You will do that by investigating your strengths of personality. This is because our values speak of what we hold most dear in the world, and that in turn is typically related to our strengths of character.

We can learn something about our strengths of character from the Values in Action Institute on Character, which is online at http://www.viacharacter.org/. The Institute is a highly respected nonprofit organization devoted to the scientific understanding of character. Their free VIA survey is designed to tell you what your main character strengths are.

Your exercise begins with reading about the VIA Institute on their website and then taking their online survey, to which the website has a link. As of this writing, almost immediately after you complete the survey, you are provided with a free readout and explanation of your character strengths as measured by your responses.

Once you have your results, reflect on what they say about your beliefs about what is most worthwhile. Make a list of the values that you believe are most fully your own. Evaluate how well those values align with your strengths of character. Then ask yourself in what ways and to what degree you feel you are living up to your strengths and your values.

This is also a good exercise on which to compare notes with a close relative or friend. Ask that person to also take the survey and get the results. Then compare notes. Do you both agree that the survey results are truly descriptive of each of you? Use the opportunity to discuss your personalities, how close the results are to how you perceive yourselves and each other, and how well your character strengths reflect your values.

Exercise 2: *Understand which Spiritual Principles Speak Most Eloquently to You*

The 12 spiritual principles set forth in this book promote not only spiritual wellness but also physical, psychological, and social well-being. This exercise asks you to consider those spiritual principles and address the question of which ones speak most eloquently and forcefully to you, and why. It is another ranking exercise since it asks you to classify the spiritual principles into three groups: most meaningful to you, second most meaningful, and third most meaningful.

Similar to the other ranking exercises you have done, the purpose of this one is to challenge you to consciously entertain each spiritual principle and how it affects or might affect your life. It's a good way to embed the principles into your thoughts so they can better guide your actions. As you do this exercise, I encourage you to read again about any of the principles that may need refreshing in your thoughts.

Once you have categorized the principles into three levels of meaningfulness to you, then for each group ask yourself to what degree you have been practicing those principles, as well as which ones you want most to practice in the future and to what degree. Then ask yourself, for each one, just how you are going to do that.

Summary of the Essences of the 12 Principles

Principle of Ayurveda: *Balance your inner nature with outer nature.*

Principle of Calmness: *Find ways to deal effectively with chronic stress: reframe the situation, accept what is, meditate; but most of all, embrace Spirit.*

Principle of Acceptance: *Do not emotionally oppose the River of Life; accept it and use its flow to power your own life.*

Principle of Thought: *Make thought your powerful ally.*

Principle of Dharma: *Find and follow your passion and purpose.*

Principle of the Virtues of Heart: *For maximum wellness and spirituality, practice the Virtues of Heart—love, friendship, compassion, and kindness.*

Principle of Harmony: *Seek harmony in all dimensions through self-knowledge.*

Principle of Seva: *Give of yourself for the well-being of others, and let the giving be your only reward.*

Principle of Now: *Embrace the wondrous Now, which is all that ever exists.*

Principle of Gratitude: *Shower the world and its many blessings with gratitude.*

Principle of the Divine You: *Recognize that Spirit abides in you, and in each of us.*

Principle of Non-Attachment: *Live a spiritual life; intend what you want, but don't become emotionally attached to it; don't let what you don't have interfere with the enjoyment of what you do have, which is great wealth and many blessings.*

About Dr. Raj

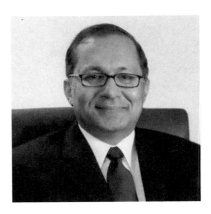

Rajiv Parti, M.D. (aka Dr. Raj) is a world-leading specialist in pain management with over thirty years of clinical practicing experience. As the Chief of Anesthesiology at Bakersfield Heart Hospital in California he specialized in cardiac anesthesia for fifteen years. Dr. Parti founded the Pain Management Institute of California in Bakersfield, and under his direction it has served thousands of patients seeking relief from acute and chronic pain.

In 2005 he personally encountered the first of a series of life-threatening health challenges that led him to explore the evidence of non-traditional treatments based on complementary and alternative medicine. His discovery of Ayurveda and his subsequent education, training, and personal practice of it have given him the rigorous academic and scientific qualifications that he was trained to look for as an allopathic doctor.

His studies and experience in this field led him to formulate an integrative approach to total wellness, especially in the areas of pain management and disorders of stress, addiction, and depression, to combine the best and most practical applications of both modern medicine and the medical care charted in the ancient wisdom traditions of India and the East. He now specializes in promoting spiritual wellness and personal growth with various non-traditional healing modalities.

Dr. Parti has worked with and been in dialogue with some of the world's most esteemed researchers in the fields of psychiatry, neuroscience, sleep medicine, and pain management from Harvard, UCSD, Berkeley, and The Scripps Center for Integrative Medicine who advocate the use of meditation, yoga, mantra (sound healing), and mandala (color therapy) for contemporary disorders.

Dr. Parti stepped down from full time clinical practice in 2010 to concentrate on his own recovery from chronic pain and to write about his findings and discoveries. Since 2012 he has been working with his colleagues at The Pain Management Institute of California researching the effect of meditation and yoga on the narcotic requirement for pain management.